WHEN SEX IS THE SUBJECT

WHEN SEX IS THE SUBJECT

ATTITUDES AND ANSWERS FOR YOUNG CHILDREN

Pamela M. Wilson, MSW

Suggestions for teachers, parents and other care providers of children to age 10

Network Publications, a division of ETR Associates
Santa Cruz, CA
1991

© 1991 by Network Publications, a division of ETR Associates.
All rights reserved. Published by Network Publications,
P.O. Box 1830, Santa Cruz, CA 95061-1830.

10 9 8 7 6 5 4 3 2

Printed in the United States of America

Illustrations by Marcia Quackenbush
Design by Julia Chiapella

Library of Congress Cataloging-in-Publication Data

Wilson, Pamela (Pamela M.)
    When Sex Is the Subject : attitudes and answers for young children : suggestions for teachers, parents and other care providers of children to age 10 / Pamela M. Wilson.
       p. cm.
    Includes bibliographical references.
    ISBN 1-56071-064-0
    1. Sex Instruction—United States. 2. Children and sex—United States. I. Title.
HQ56.W648   1991
372.3'72—dc20   91-739
                                                 CIP

Title No. 583

This book is dedicated to my dear friend and colleague, Mary Lee Tatum, whose pioneering work in sexuality education has influenced me profoundly and will live on through the efforts of countless others.

—*PMW*

Contents

Acknowledgments ix

Introduction   The Concept of Music: The Importance of Attitudes in Sexuality Education   1
How Do Children Learn About Sexuality?   2
Hazardous Messages About Sexuality   4
Starting Early to Promote Positive Attitudes   5
How to Use This Book   6

Chapter 1.   How Children Learn They Are Sexual People   9
How Children Grow and Change Psychologically and Socially   10
  Birth to Age Two   10
  Ages Three and Four   10
  Ages Five to Eight   11
  Ages Nine to Twelve   12
How Children Think and Process Information   13
  Birth to Age Two   13
  Ages Three and Four   14
  Ages Five to Eight   15
  Ages Nine to Twelve   15
How Children Develop Sexual Identity   16

Chapter 2.   Responding to Children at Their Own Level   21
Taking Off Adult Glasses   22
Making Abstract Ideas Concrete   28

Chapter 3.   Answering Children's Questions: Guidelines, Tips and
              Suggestions   33
              General Guidelines to Keep in Mind   34
              What About Personal Questions?   36
              A Question of Values   37
              Examples of Questions and Answers   39
                  Preschool Through First Grade Questions   39
                  Second and Third Grade Questions   41
                  Fourth and Fifth Grade Questions   43

Chapter 4.   Especially for Teachers: Sexuality Education in the
              Classroom   49
              Goals of Planned Sexuality Education   50
              Special Concerns About Teaching Sexuality to Young Children   52
              Training Teachers to Be Prepared   53
              Creating a Positive Learning Environment   55
              Handling Group Discussions: The Question Box   58
              Teaching About Sexual Abuse   62
              When the Teacher Is a Man   64
              Teachers Learning About Parents   65
              Parents and Teachers as Partners Providing Sexuality Education   66

Chapter 5.   Especially for Parents: Sexuality Education at Home   69
              What Do Parents Worry About?   70
              Important Messages for Parents About Sexuality   79

Appendix A.   Sexuality Concepts in Concrete Terms   81
Appendix B.   Organizations Involved in Sexuality Education   85
Appendix C.   Books for Professionals, Parents and Children   89
References   101

Acknowledgments

I'd like to express my appreciation to the many friends and colleagues who supported and guided me during the process of writing this book. My multitalented friend Terry Quinn helped me conceptualize the basic themes, gave me valuable advice about writing style and did the initial editing. Jean Hunter, a major force behind my work with elementary teachers, assisted in a myriad of ways including keeping me abreast of changing issues in elementary family life education programs.

Peggy Brick, Mary Lee Tatum and Jane Quinn generously read the first draft and made many useful comments. Claire Sholtz gave me valuable input, shared curriculum materials and distributed surveys to teachers in Irvington, New Jersey. Thanks to the many teachers from Irvington who took the time to complete the surveys.

I'd like to acknowledge Winnie Bayard, Debra Haffner, Deborah Wilson Haul, Linda Watson, my nephews Brian and Evin, and all the other parents and children with whom I've worked over the years who have contributed to my knowledge base and repertoire of anecdotes.

I'd also like to thank the elementary teachers I've trained, especially those in Alexandria, Virginia, who have taught me so much about educating young children. Special thanks to Beth Cronin, Pam Walkup, Brenda Alexander, Priscilla Douglas, Carole Freeman, Carolyn Holland, Cici Jukoski, and Ellen Killalea.

Finally, it's been a pleasure to work with Kay Clark, my editor at ETR Associates, who has provided wisdom, inspiration, patience and support throughout the entire process.

Introduction

The Concept of Music: The Importance of Attitudes in Sexuality Education

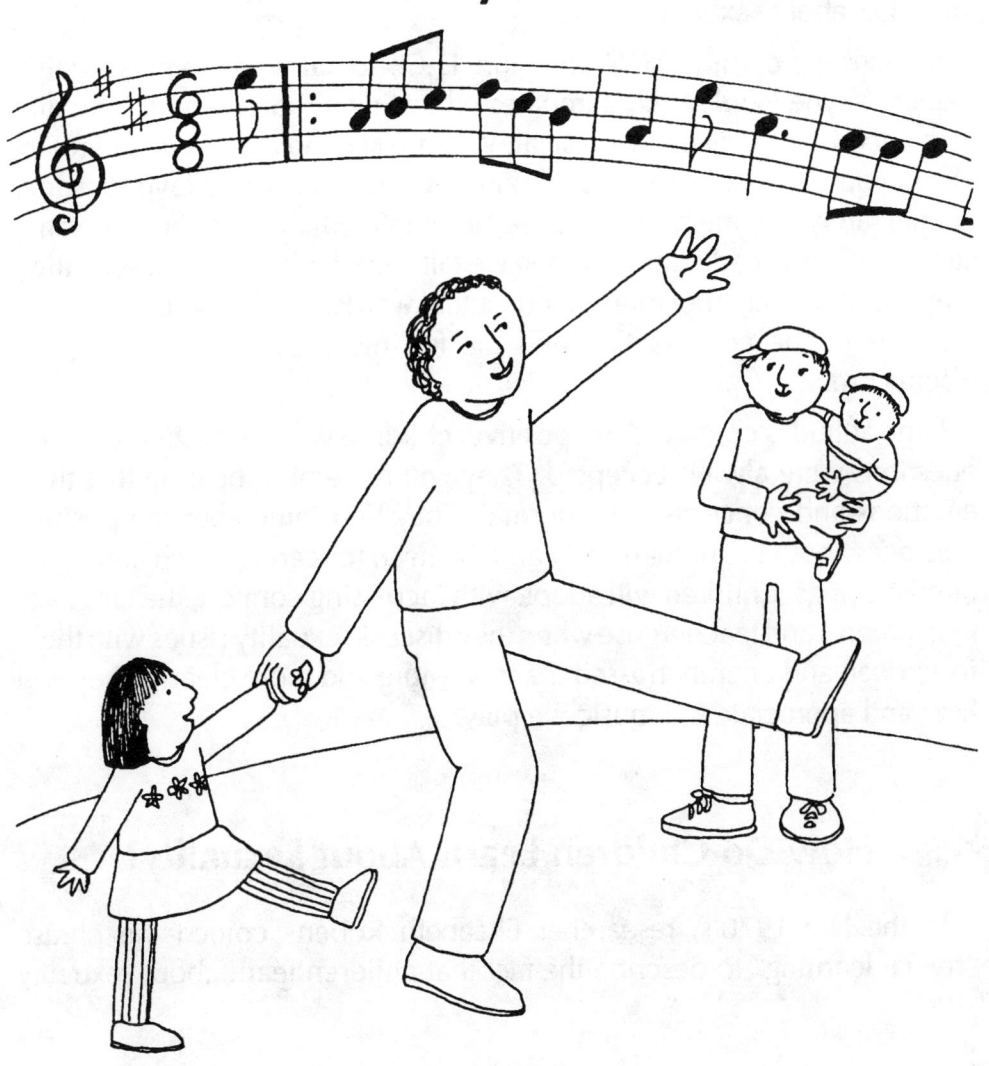

Throughout the years, several key people have influenced my ideas about the concept of "music" in sexuality education. Michael Carrera, nationally renowned author, educator and trainer, talks about the need to "keep a broad definition of sexuality in front of you all the time." Dr. Carrera believes that society has performed a "sexectomy" on the true nature of human sexuality by narrowing the focus to include little more than genital sex. He stresses that the words we use to educate children about sexuality are not nearly as important as the "music" we play. In other words, it is not so much what we say but how we say it that provides children with healthy messages about sexuality.

A colleague of mine in Washington, D.C., social worker and sexuality trainer Wayne Pawlowski, compares educating children about sexuality with attending a Broadway musical. When you go to a musical and really like it, you often leave the show humming the melody of a favorite song. People rarely sing the lyrics because they can't remember them. The same can be true in sex education. When we talk with children about sexuality, they may not remember many of our actual words, but they will remember the tone of the conversation and the feelings engendered during the discussion.

If the attitudes conveyed are positive, children will remember that their questions were always accepted. They will remember hearing that their emotions and concerns were normal. They will remember the positive messages about the human body and the need for caring touch among all human beings. Children will adopt, with increasing comfort, the language their parents and teachers use when they discuss sexuality issues with them in an open and unembarrassed manner. More and more clearly, they will hear and appreciate the music we play.

How Do Children Learn About Sexuality?

In the late 1970's, researcher Elizabeth Roberts coined the phrase "sexual learning" to describe the fact that children learn about sexuality every day of their lives regardless of what parents, teachers or other adults do or don't tell them. They learn not only by listening to adults but by observing them: the way they interact with other people; the way they show (or fail to show) affection; their reaction to TV programs and events in the community; and the attitudes they convey in their conversations with other adults.

Children also learn about sexuality from the media—children's TV programs, afternoon soap operas, morning talk shows, evening sitcoms, news shows, movies, print ads, teen magazines, music videos and commercials. According to Nielson Media Research, the average American family has a television set turned on over seven hours each day. At the same time, children are constantly picking up information—and misinformation—from their friends in the form of jokes, casual talk and attitude-revealing behavior.

Let's look more closely at what children are learning. Messages from parents or caretakers vary from home to home. Some families show affection openly, others do not. Some parents are comfortable with nudity, take baths with their children, skinny dip together and so on. Others may not engage in such activities with their children but aren't uncomfortable if their children find them nude in the bathroom or the bedroom. Still other parents show displeasure if their children catch even a glimpse of them nude.

Media messages are loaded with sexual content. Children's cartoons, and more importantly, commercials during cartoon hours, give definite messages about gender role behavior—how boys and girls should act, appropriate toys for boys and girls, and so on. Researchers have found that there are as many as 20,000 scenes of suggested sexual intercourse and behavior, sexual comment and innuendo in a year of prime-time television. Adult TV programming, not intended for young children but often watched by them, is filled with messages—some clear, some ambiguous; some sensitive, some irresponsible—about male/female relationships, transsexualism, transvestism, teenage pregnancy, homosexuality, rape, sexual abuse and other topics about which children are naturally curious.

The Concept of Music

Hazardous Messages About Sexuality

Today's children are growing up in an era plagued by social problems related to sexuality. There is greater awareness of child sexual abuse; the problem of teenage pregnancy has not gone away; and now AIDS has made death a potential consequence of unsafe sexual behavior.

Today's children are dating at younger ages and having sex at younger ages. In some urban communities the average age that boys report beginning sexual intercourse is 12. In light of these sobering realities, many school and community programs have focused on "disaster prevention"—educational efforts designed to help children avoid specific sexuality-related problems. Thus some states mandate AIDS education without providing any sexuality education. Many primary classrooms offer child sexual abuse prevention, though often not in the context of a broader discussion of family life and sexuality.

This sexual learning environment is potentially hazardous for children. What message would you get about sex if the only thing you were told in formal settings was that some adults force children to have sex and that sex can lead to AIDS? Sexuality educators worry that a great many of today's young generation will grow up to be anxiety-ridden, sexually dysfunctional adults.

In my work teaching elementary school children and training elementary school teachers, I have learned that many children come to school with preformed attitudes, both positive and negative, about sexuality. Some families have tried hard to raise their children in nonsexist ways and to present sexuality as a normal topic of conversation. However, a wide range of factors influence every child's socialization.

For reasons that go well beyond parental instruction or modeling, *some* children learn early that:

- Sex is a taboo topic.
- The human body is shameful.
- The genitals are nasty.
- Roles for boys and girls are rigidly determined.

Teachers often find that children giggle when sexuality is discussed in the classroom, especially as students approach third and fourth grades. The giggling can be a sign that children are internalizing society's confused and often negative attitudes about the topic.

A teacher I had trained once phoned me very upset. He had shown a film entitled "Human and Animal Beginnings" to his third grade class. After portraying the birth of various kinds of animals, the film showed a brief shot of a human baby being born. The baby's head was shown emerging from the mother's vagina. Afterwards the children asked, "Did our parents know we were going to see this film? Were we supposed to see that? Was that X-rated?" What messages had these children picked up about the female genitals? Clearly they had learned somewhere that the vagina, in and of itself, even in the process of childbirth, was pornographic. What a frightening attitude to instill in young children.

Starting Early to Promote Positive Attitudes

Societal norms and values about sexuality can and do influence children's attitudes about themselves—how comfortable they are with their own bodies, how they think they should behave as boys or girls, how comfortable they are with physical affection, whether they view themselves as attractive. Societal biases also influence how children view and treat others.

The National Association for the Education of Young Children reports that children as young as three "exhibit 'pre-prejudice' toward others on the basis of gender or race or being differently-abled" and that by age five they use racial reasons for refusing to interact with children different from themselves (Derman-Sparks and the A.B.C. Task Force, 1989). Certainly by fourth grade children become masters at name-calling, with "gay" and "fag" leading the list of universal put-downs.

The earlier parents and educators begin to consciously plan the messages we give young children, the greater the likelihood we can encourage

The Concept of Music

their sense of themselves as lovable, capable and responsible sexual beings, and the greater the possibility that children will approach diversity among human beings with comfort and empathy.

Little has been written about ways to address sexuality issues with young children. The few books that have done so have been targeted primarily to parents. Yet, program planners and educators are also searching for appropriate content for the primary grades. Educators who talk freely with adolescents about sensitive issues often get nervous when faced with the challenge of discussing sexuality with four to ten year olds. They may wonder, "What will I say to these children? How will they react? Am I putting ideas in their heads? Will their parents object?"

Many parents have similar worries: "When should I bring up the subject of sex with my children? What should or shouldn't I say? I know I shouldn't react negatively when my daughter touches her genitals, but it upsets me. I caught my son pretending to have sex with another child...what should I do? How can I protect my child from AIDS?"

These are all valid questions and concerns. Parents and educators want to keep children safe from emotional and physical harm. The challenge in sexuality education is to arm children with the information, attitudes and skills that they need to keep themselves safe from abuse, unplanned pregnancy and disease and, at the same time, help them develop the capacity for adult sexual relationships that are loving, healthy and responsible.

This book will help you think about both the words and the music to the songs we play for children. We will compose the melodies and the lyrics and identify practical strategies for delivering appropriate sexuality messages to children.

How to Use This Book

There are five chapters in this book. Chapter 1 presents basic information about sexual development in children. It offers insights into they way children think about, understand and experience their sexuality from birth through age 12.

Chapter 2 gives parents and educators a window into the child's view of sexuality. It will help you distinguish between adult and childhood sexuality and presents guidelines for "starting where children are" and responding to them at their own level. It also offers strategies for making abstract ideas about sexuality more concrete for young children. You'll discover ways to create simple explanations that convey positive "music."

Chapter 3 gives general guidelines for answering children's questions and sample questions and answers for three age groups: preschool through first grade, second and third grade, and fourth and fifth grade.

Chapter 4 gives specific advice to teachers of young children. It identifies the goals of sex education, the need for adequate training, ways to create a positive climate for discussing sexuality, methods for handling group discussion, responses to teachers' common concerns and suggestions for developing effective partnerships with parents.

Chapter 5 gives specific advice to parents. It clarifies the important role parents play as transmitters of values and presents a strategy for correctly interpreting your children's behavior and responding in a manner that conveys your specific point of view about sexuality. In this chapter you'll also find sample questions and answers as well as a list of important messages that are intended to guide and reassure you as you begin or continue the important process of sexuality education with your sons and daughters.

The terms "educator" and "teacher" are used interchangeably throughout the book. The two terms refer to anyone who teaches young children, and are not meant to be limited to those who teach in a classroom setting.

There are many ways that different audiences can make use of this book:

- Parents might read it from cover to cover to get helpful advice for understanding and dealing with their own children, or they might keep it around as a resource to consult when a difficult situation or question arises.

- People who are new to the field of sexuality education can gain insight into its philosophical approach, format, techniques and content.
- Primary and elementary school teachers can get ideas for incorporating sexuality information and attitudes into their ongoing curriculum.
- Both new and experienced educators can enhance specific skills, especially in the areas of answering questions, promoting positive attitudes and presenting information simply.
- Trainers and administrators can find ideas and content for workshops with teachers and parents.
- Administrators might also use the book as a starting point for the development of a sexuality education program for young children in their schools or community agencies.

Chapter 1

How Children Learn They Are Sexual People

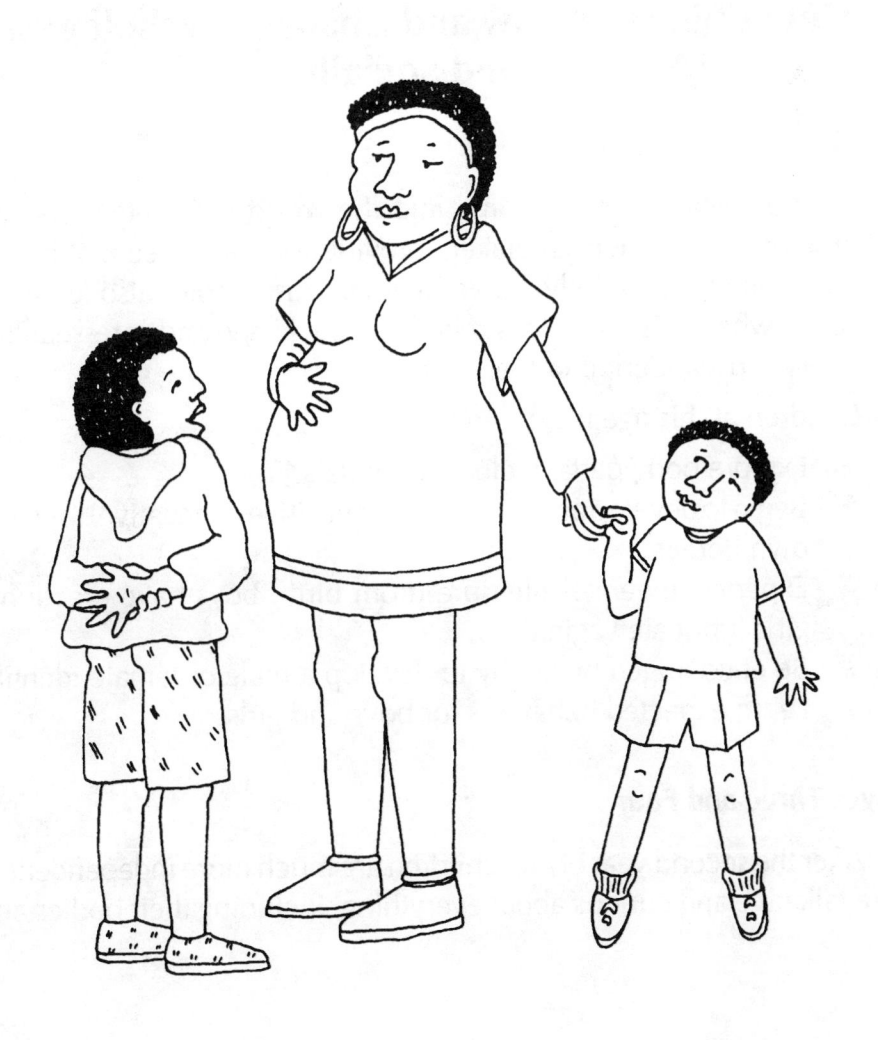

From the moment of birth, children begin learning about themselves as sexual people. The concept of *development* is very helpful in understanding how all of us see and experience the world at different points in our lives. As children grow physically, their abilities, their thinking patterns, their attention spans, their feelings, and a host of other characteristics change and develop in recognizable ways. This chapter will examine three areas of human growth and development that have relevance for sexuality education: psychosocial, cognitive and sexual.

How Children Grow and Change Psychologically and Socially

Birth to Age Two

Psychologically, infants come into the world completely dependent. They require that their caretakers provide for every need. When those needs are met consistently, babies learn to trust. Babies also learn how to be loved when they are held, stroked, patted, kissed and caressed. Infancy is a very sensual period of life.

Children at this age may:

- Explore body parts, including genitals.
- Begin to develop an attitude (either positive or negative) toward their own bodies.
- Experience genital pleasure (from birth, boys have erections and girls lubricate vaginally).
- Be encouraged by family to develop a male or female identity.
- Learn expected behaviors for boys and girls.

Ages Three and Four

After the second year of life, children are much more independent. They are talkative and curious about everything, including their bodies and the bodies of others. It is common to see three year olds peeking under one another's clothing, undressing their dolls, and checking out the "bottoms" of pets and stuffed animals. By this age boys know they have a penis, which they handle to urinate. Girls are rarely taught about the analogous part of their bodies, the clitoris.

In *The Touch Film* (Sterling Productions), psychologist Jesse Potter says that boys want to know why their penises are called privates. She points out that in reality boys have "publics" and girls have "privates." After all, boys see and touch their penises everyday, use urinals openly in public bathrooms and typically observe each other naked in locker rooms. Girls' genitals are much more secret. They can't even *see* their own vulvas without making a conscious effort, and most girls don't find out that they have a clitoris until well beyond the childhood years.

Children at this age may:

- Become aware of and very curious about gender/body differences.
- Masturbate unless taught not to.
- Play house, doctor or explore other forms of sex play with friends and siblings.
- Establish a firm internal belief that they are either male or female.
- Have fun with bathroom humor.
- Mimic adult sexual behavior.
- Begin to repeat curse words.
- Be curious about their own origins: "Where did I come from?"

Ages Five to Eight

Children in this age group have moved into the world beyond home and have begun to find their place in it. They realize they are starting to be judged on their own rather than their family's merits. They begin to reorganize the way they see themselves and the way they behave to adapt to new social situations. Children bring varying levels of knowledge and skill to this period of life depending on their family and preschool experiences.

Children at this age may:
- Continue sex play and masturbation.
- Be very curious about pregnancy and birth.
- Have strong same-sex friendships. Girls and boys learn different styles of communicating. Girls tend to form close intimate friendships with one or two other girls. Boys usually play in larger groups; their play is rougher and more oriented around mutual interests in activities (Maccoby, 1990).
- Show strong interest in male/female roles that are often stereotyped, regardless of parents' approach to childrearing.
- Have a basic sexual orientation by this time.
- Have a new awareness of authority figures—teachers may be seen as knowing more than parents.
- Compare their own situations with those of peers; complain about lack of fairness.
- Begin to conform with peer group style of dress and speech. At this age boys experience more pressure than girls to adhere to sex-role expectations in areas such as choice of toys, hobbies, clothing and hair styles.
- Engage in name-calling and teasing.

Ages Nine to Twelve

For many children, especially girls, fourth or fifth grade marks the onset of puberty. At this age, children are intensely curious, constantly teasing and interested in everything. At the early end of this stage, they approach sexuality information in a direct and scientific manner. However, since girls tend to mature faster than boys, they often seem to feel more nervous and to act more secretively during discussions about puberty, probably because the whole topic is closer to them than it is for boys.

Most children are very interested in music, clothes and all that it takes to be "cool." Some even have a "boyfriend" or "girlfriend" whom they see at school and talk to on the phone.

Children at this age may:
- Enter puberty, especially girls. Early pubertal development is perceived positively by most boys but negatively by many girls.
- Become more modest and desire privacy.
- Experience emotional ups and downs.
- Develop romantic crushes on friends, older teens, music and TV idols, or sometimes teachers and counselors.
- Continue to attach importance to same sex friends.
- Feel awkward and wonder "Am I normal?"
- Masturbate to orgasm.
- Be strongly influenced by peer group, but parents remain the major source of values.
- Continue to learn society's expectations about appropriate behavior for boys and girls. Girls, more than boys, experience increased pressure to conform to stereotyped sex roles. They may avoid academic achievement, for example, preferring to base their popularity on appearance, personality or possessions.
- Begin to penetrate the mysteries of the adult world by using sexual language and enjoying romantic and sexual fantasies.
- Face decisions about sex and drugs.
- Initiate sexual intercourse as early as age 12.

How Children Think and Process Information

Birth to Age Two

For about the first 18 months, a child perceives the world very literally. Infants can only digest what they can see, hear or touch at a given moment. They're learning to pay attention to the information that comes in through each of their senses. In her classic book, *The Magic Years,* Selma Fraiberg refers to the concept of the "vanishing object." When Daddy displays a toy to his six month old and then hides the toy behind his back, the baby thinks the toy is gone. If the baby can't see it, it's not there. Babies perceive everything happening around them to be the result of their own actions. If they pull a toy, it moves. If they close their eyes, the world goes blank—like magic.

By 10 to 12 months of age, children begin to know that a toy can be hidden from sight but still exist. By the end of this period, most children have developed some language. They delight in pointing to and labeling parts of the body.

Ages Three and Four

Children at this age are still concrete thinkers but they are making progress. They are beginning to realize that there is a world outside of themselves. They might begin to engage in symbolic play, such as pretending to call Auntie, who lives in a different house. For our purposes, though, we must realize that children have difficulty understanding ideas that have not been a part of their direct experience. So in trying to make sense of things like sex and birth, three and four year olds are likely to create theories that relate to what they themselves have seen, heard or felt.

For example, in seeing a pregnant woman (a woman with a "fat stomach"), the child guesses that the woman has eaten something to make her stomach fat. Or the child might guess that the baby had existed someplace else and got magically placed inside the mother's body. When we tell children about reproduction, they don't always accept our theories because these theories just don't make sense to them in the context of their own experiences.

Anne Bernstein conducted research with children to find out how they understood information about reproduction and birth at different ages. In her book, *The Flight of the Stork,* Bernstein labels children in this age group "the geographers," because their theories focus on where the baby has come from (the store, Mom's tummy or the hospital). Geographers believe the baby has always existed and for some reason has now come to live in their family.

Some four year olds may have reached the next level of understanding—manufacturing—in which the child guesses that babies are manufactured by people in the same way cars are produced in a factory. "Manufacturers" create stories to explain how the baby was made, such as the mother eats something that grows inside her tummy. Understanding that children think this way makes it clear that using language like "the father plants his seed in the mother" only further confirms the child's mythical thinking.

Mythical thinking about sex and reproduction is developmentally appropriate and not harmful. However, our goal is to help children move beyond the myths—not to further reinforce them. We must be patient, though, and recognize that children can be persistent in holding on to their own theories in the face of new factual information.

Ages Five to Eight

This is a time of enormous cognitive growth as a child moves slowly toward abstract thought. By age six or seven most children are beginning to understand generalizations that go beyond their concrete experiences. For example, in explaining why we have laws, a seven year old might say, "So people won't get hurt." These children are learning not to be fooled by physical appearances. They can learn, for example, that 2+5=7 is the same as 7=5+2. Five to eight year olds are active learners concerned with how things work and how they're made. Their ideas are starting to be strongly influenced not only by what they see and hear but by what they read.

Bernstein sees this stage as a transitional period in a child's understanding of reproduction. Children in this age group may be able to recite the basic facts about reproduction but they don't quite grasp the full story. Maybe they know the mother's egg meets with the father's sperm, but they think the egg is large and has a shell. They may know that it takes a man and a woman to make a baby but perhaps they think the man and woman have to be married for reproduction to occur.

Ages Nine to Twelve

This is a time when children practice the skills they've been learning. At this age they are completely open to new information. For this reason, many family life educators enjoy working with them. However, even

How Children Learn They Are Sexual People

though children are taking in the information, they aren't yet thinking very deeply about the new ideas. Adults can help by setting up time for reflection after each new experience or learning activity.

We can challenge the literal thinking of fourth, fifth and sixth graders by asking open-ended questions such as "What would you do if..." and "What would happen if...." In fact, children this age ask many of their own questions that way: "What happens when a boy and girl have sex at an early age?" or "What would happen if a lady was having three babies, was in an airplane crash and her stomach got hurt?"

Bernstein labels the next two levels of children's understanding "concrete physiology" and "preformation." Concrete physiologists can consider past, present and future, and understand cause and effect. It's clear to them that sexual intercourse is the vehicle for bringing together the sperm and the egg, but these little scientists aren't sure why it's necessary for the two cells to unite. Children who believe in preformation think the fetus already exists in either the sperm or the egg, and that the connection between the two cells is only needed to promote the growth of the pre-existing fetus.

According to Bernstein, it isn't until around age 12 that most children can really put the story of reproduction together completely. Ironically, this is also the average age that boys in some urban communities say that they have intercourse for the first time (Clark, Zabin and Hardy, 1984).

How Children Develop Sexual Identity

The final area of development has to do with children's growing awareness of themselves as sexual persons—male or female—who are attracted to other people—male and/or female. There are four issues to consider here: biosexual identity, core gender identity, gender role identity and sexual orientation.

Biosexual Identity

Each child comes into the world with genitals, reproductive organs, genes and hormones—a physiological package that is biologically determined and not influenced by the culture.

Core Gender Identity

This refers to a person's internal sense of being either male or female. Up until around 18 months of age, children don't know for sure whether they're boys or girls. They learn their gender by the way they're labeled by others and by their own observations. Girls observe that they have bodies like their mothers, aunts, or perhaps their sisters. "I am like mother. Mother is a female. So I must be female."

Somewhere between 18 months and three years of age, children develop a strong internal conviction that they're either male or female. Usually their conviction matches their physical package, but sometimes it doesn't and then confusion, isolation and discomfort can follow.

Gender Role Identity

Gender role identity refers to children's adopting specific behaviors that their culture says are appropriate for them as boys or girls. A child's gender role identity is influenced by many factors, including personality, education, family and culture.

Strong cultural messages about how boys should behave and how girls should behave begin to influence children from the time they're born. Studies have shown that parents and other adults behave one way with boys and another way with girls.

Sexual Orientation

Orientation is a term used to describe a person's potential for romantic and sexual attraction to others. Some people are oriented toward members of the same sex, some toward the other sex, and others toward both sexes.

Popular theories about sexual orientation suggest that the majority of us have the potential to be romantically and sexually attracted to both sexes. Few people are either exclusively homosexual or exclusively heterosexual in their orientation.

Some people use the term sexual preference rather than sexual orientation. However, this term is problematic because it implies that a person chooses his or her feelings of romantic and sexual attraction to others. By and large, these feelings are not chosen. Many experts in the field now believe that orientation is determined early in life, possibly by age five, that it probably has a strong biological influence, and that it can't be changed.

There's a difference between sexual orientation and sexual behavior. A person can be oriented toward members of the same sex and never act on that attraction. Children learn early that society is prejudiced against homosexuality. Recognizing feelings of same-sex attraction is very scary for young people in our society. Gay men and lesbians often recall periods during adolescence and young adulthood when they denied their feelings to themselves and to significant others in their lives.

The important point here is that orientation and behavior are two different things. Orientation is the internal feeling of romantic and sexual attraction to others. A man can have sex with other men, or a woman with other women, and not be gay. This happens frequently in institutions where same sex people are housed together.

To further complicate these issues, there is the concept of personal identity (self-perception). How does the person actually see him- or herself—as homosexual, bisexual or heterosexual? How does the person present him or herself to friends and family? Some people are oriented toward members of the same sex, have sex only with members of the other sex, see themselves as heterosexual, and feel a great deal of conflict inside. Others are oriented toward members of the same sex, have sex with members of the same sex, but have not acknowledged to themselves or the world that they are gay or lesbian. Of course, there are many men and women who have recognized their sexual orientation, behave in accordance with it and identify comfortably as gay men or lesbians.

Sorting out the Confusion: Identity, Orientation, Roles

In my work with teens and adults in educational programs, I've seen people struggle with several confusing issues. First, people often confuse gender identity with sexual orientation. I've heard both youth and adults remark that a lesbian is a woman who wants to be a man: "Why else would she want to have sex with a woman?" For the most part, lesbians and gay men have a gender identity that matches their physical make-up. Gay men see themselves as men, but they're attracted to other men. Lesbians are comfortable with themselves as women, yet they find themselves loving other women.

People may also confuse role identity with sexual orientation. They think men who behave in ways considered to be "feminine" are probably gay or have "tendencies" in that direction. Women who compete competitively in organized sports or who coach athletic teams are often labeled as lesbians. Homosexuality is not caused by an individual's adoption of roles or characteristics commonly associated with the other gender. An "effeminate" man can be homosexual, bisexual or heterosexual.

Confusion about these issues, combined with fear of homosexuality, can contribute to the kind of sex-role stereotyping that's limiting—and at times harmful—to children. For example, a parent or teacher might discourage a child from engaging in nontraditional activities, hobbies or chores, thinking that such behaviors will encourage homosexuality. Then the child misses out on experiences that could be enjoyable and personally fulfilling.

Chapter 2

Responding to Children at Their Own Level

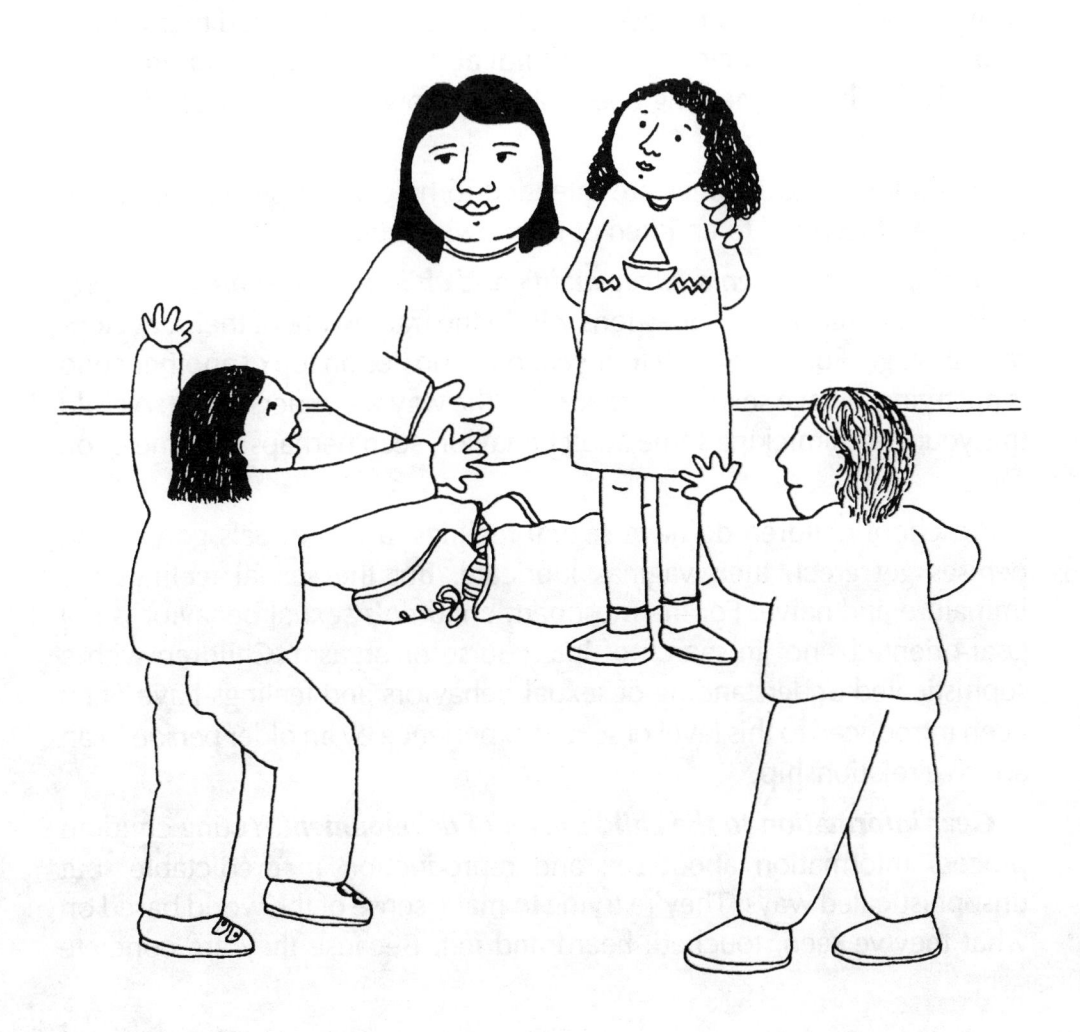

The last chapter reviewed background information about children's development. This chapter uses that information to shape a set of guidelines for teaching young children about sexuality and influencing their sexual development in positive ways.

Taking Off Adult Glasses

One of the biggest challenges adults face as we take on this important task is getting into the mind set of children. Our perception of sexuality is completely different from that of children because we've had many more years to internalize societal and cultural attitudes. In fact children might actually teach us something about attitudes toward sex because of their fresh perspective.

The following guidelines are intended to help you take off your adult glasses and respond to children at their own level.

Distinguish between adult sexuality and childhood sexuality. Interpret children's behavior and questions within the framework of their developmental stage. For example, a four year old who lies on top of another child is not trying to have sexual intercourse in the way we understand it. A child this young is mimicking some adult behavior, seen perhaps at home or on TV.

Preschool children do have sexual feelings: a touch feels good, their penises get erect, their vaginas lubricate. But the sexual feelings are immature and naive. For the most part, children's sexual behavior is not goal-oriented—not in search of intercourse or orgasm. Children with a sophisticated understanding of sexual behaviors and feelings have often been introduced to this level of sexual experience by an older person in an abusive relationship.

Gear information to the child's level of development. Young children process information about sex and reproduction in predictable, but unsophisticated ways. They're trying to make sense of the world based on what they've seen, touched, heard and felt. Because they are concrete thinkers, children are most concerned with the where, what and how of reproduction. Where does the baby come from? How is the baby made? Where was the baby before it was born? Children create theories to answer these questions, sometimes preferring their own myths to our correct but hard-to-believe explanations.

Ask questions to find out children's current understanding of an issue. Then give information that will nudge them onto the next level of understanding. Some adults worry, "What if I give a child too much information? Will knowing the names of sexual parts of the body lead to a loss of innocence? Will knowing about sexual intercourse cause my child to want to try it? Will information overwhelm the child?" There aren't simple answers to these questions. We should naturally avoid giving children information beyond their level of understanding. However, the most likely danger in giving children sexuality information they can't understand is in boring them. Elementary teachers will attest to the fact that children typically ignore information that is "over their heads."

Explicit sexual messages that can be stressful for children usually come not from conversations at school or at home but from watching TV, movies and music videos. Today's environment of sexual learning is quite provocative, increasing children's need for guidance and direction from the responsible adults in their lives. That is why sexuality education in schools is so important.

Less is better than more. This advice has been very helpful to the primary teachers I've trained. It simply means that when dealing with four, five and six year olds, you should begin with the simplest explanation (what I call the "less answer") and move on to a more complicated explanation if the children continue to be interested or keep asking questions. Because it's such a challenge to get out of the adult mind set, parents and teachers frequently fall into the trap of giving far too complicated answers to children's questions.

In dealing with very young children, the best response is sometimes just to give a name to something. If a four year old sees a sanitary napkin and asks, "What is that?", avoid the urge to talk about uteruses, eggs or blood.

When I posed this question to a group of parents roleplaying at a workshop, the group squirmed with anxiety. Finally, a brave mother responded to the "child" by saying, "That's a sanitary napkin." The other parents were amazed by the simplicity and beauty of that response, which is one that would satisfy most young children. If the child is not satisfied and continues to ask questions, the adult should continue to answer.

Approach sexuality issues proactively rather than reactively. Children need guidance from adults to prepare them for each stage of psychological, social and sexual development. The focus of our interactions with children should be on their positive development as sexual human beings, not simply on helping them avoid sexual abuse or teenage pregnancy. It is understandable that educators, parents, agencies and funders want to reduce problems related to sexuality. But a focus on "disaster prevention" sidetracks us from the true goal of sexuality education, which is to give children the information, attitudes and skills they need to become healthy and responsible sexual adults.

Keep the door open for communication. This means saying and doing things to let children know you're open to talking about sexuality, that you welcome questions and comments. In her book on parent-child communication, *What Do You Say After You Clear Your Throat?*, Jean Gochros tells parents that they should institute what she calls an "opening doors policy" with their children. Gochros says:

> "A true open door policy means that you actively open the doors, keep on opening them, and when the child opens the doors, you open them even wider. Door openers are useful not only because of any discussion of factual information given at the moment, but because they provide information about attitudes and pave the way for future questions."

How does an adult institute an opening doors policy? There are many small things you can do on a regular basis, such as paying close attention to comments children make. For example, a six year old might say, "Girls can't play basketball," or "Shenika's going to have a new baby at her house."

Adults have several options available to them when children make such comments:

- Ignore them.
- "Close the door" with a shocked, disapproving or angry remark.
- "Open the door" by asking a related question, smiling, nodding or otherwise encouraging the child to continue, or by making a positive statement about what the child has just said.

Here are some door-opening techniques:

- Watch for children's nonverbal cues of interest and curiosity.
- Answer questions immediately and calmly with a friendly and open facial expression.
- Bring up sexuality issues in response to events going on at home, in the neighborhood or on TV.
- Discuss sexuality issues with older children when younger children are within earshot.
- Avoid long, technical lectures and feel free to use your sense of humor as a way of easing natural tension or embarrassment.

Set up opportunities for children to learn through observation and to discover things for themselves. Here are some examples:

- Conduct bathroom tours to demystify boys' and girls' bathrooms.
- Provide opportunities for play with anatomically-correct dolls, playhouses and clothing for dress-up.
- When reading with children, include books that deal with sexuality topics (see Appendix C).
- Provide experiences with pregnant women and babies.
- See to it that children are exposed to families from diverse backgrounds.

Create an anti-bias environment in your home or classroom. Show that you value diversity in the friends or the images of people that you bring into your home or classroom. Establish a firm ground rule that makes it unacceptable to reject or tease anyone based on who he or she is as a person (black, white, poor, rich, fat, skinny, gay).

Through your words and actions, give the message that individual differences in human beings exist, are positive, and are OK to talk about. Sometimes we make young children feel they've said something wrong if they comment on another child's skin color, hair type or physical ability. These topics then become as taboo as explicit sexuality issues. It seems we need an opening doors policy for issues of diversity, too!

In their helpful pamphlet, *Teaching Young Children to Resist Bias: What Parents Can Do,* Derman-Sparks, Gutierrez and Phillips (1990) suggest ways that adults can open the door to communication. If asked, "Why is Kaseef's skin so dark?" instead of saying skin color doesn't matter, say, "His skin is dark because his parents have dark skin. We all have a special chemical in our skin that determines how dark our skin will be. If you have a little of the chemical, your skin is light. If you have a lot, your skin is dark."

Suppose your son asks, "Why does Miyoko speak funny?" Instead of hushing him up, say, "Miyoko doesn't speak funny, she speaks differently than you do. She speaks Japanese like her mom and dad. It's OK to ask questions about Miyoko, but it's not OK to say that she's funny or weird because that can hurt her feelings."

Don't forget the music. Remember, the words you use to communicate with children are important, but the music that you play (the emotional content of your words) is even more critical. Whenever possible, convey the following feelings and attitudinal messages as a part of your communication with children:

- Sexuality is a natural and positive aspect of being human.
- The human body, with all its variations and imperfections, is beautiful and good.
- The genitals are a good part of the human body.
- Everyone needs caring, nonexploitive touch.
- All individuals, including children, have the right to say who will touch them, especially on sexual parts of their bodies.
- Sex is a topic that children can and should discuss with parents, teachers, relatives and friends.
- Sexual behavior plays a role in people's lives that goes beyond

reproduction. It is also a means of showing love, experiencing pleasure and having fun.
- Sex is more than intercourse.
- Boys and girls have many similarities and a few body differences.
- Each child grows individually, at a rate that's normal for him or her.
- People's feelings are important and normal. However, one will not and should not always act on feelings.
- Stereotypes limit people in how they see themselves and others.
- Differences among human beings should be recognized and affirmed.
- It is wrong to exploit or take unfair advantage of another person.

The music you play for children can take many forms: words that convey positive feelings; relaxed and open facial expressions; quick action to stop any form of discrimination in your home or classroom; acceptance of children's honest feelings, concerns and questions; a reassuring tone of voice as you explain variations in children's development; a willingness to discuss an issue even when you feel a little embarrassed; a readiness to discuss the pleasure associated with sexual feelings and behavior as well as the negative consequences; your delight in the wonders afforded us as we experience one another through each of our senses—smell, touch, vision and hearing.

Avoid behaviors that imply negative attitudes such as:
- Frowning when children say something contrary to your beliefs or opinions.
- Discussing attitudes and feelings as if there are absolute right and wrong ways to think and feel.
- Talking children out of their feelings ("You don't or shouldn't feel that way.").
- Handling a diagram of the genitalia as if it were a smelly undershirt.
- Reinforcing stereotypes about individuals or groups of people.

Responding to Children at Their Own Level

Making Abstract Ideas Concrete

Through about age eight, children tend to depend on their knowledge and experience to process new ideas and concepts. Two psychologists who have studied this age group, Anne Bernstein and Jane Healy, recommend that adults meet children where they are in their thinking ability and then use techniques to try to bring them along to the next level of cognitive ability. This sounds great but how do you do it? Although each child and each class of students is different, the following techniques are generally useful.

Ask questions. To determine the child's current level of thinking about sex and reproduction, try asking, "Where were you before you were born?" I asked this of my nephew Evin when he was four and he answered, "In Mommy's breast." I explained that he was inside his mom but not in her breast—that he was in a special part of her body called the uterus which is down a little lower in the body than the breast. Later I learned how fond children can be of their own theories on sexuality. When I asked Evin again that same day where he was before he was born, he said, "In Mom's breast." Over the next months, though, I noticed that Evin made references to being inside his mom and asked questions about how he had gotten in and how he got out.

Use pictures and diagrams. Appropriate visuals help clarify explanations. For example, kindergarten children will have an easier time understanding physical differences between boys and girls if they can see a drawing of a boy with a penis and a girl with a vulva. Seeing is believing for young children. However, the drawings must be clear and not confusing. If you show diagrams of reproductive organs to elementary school children, make sure the organs appear within an outline of the whole body.

Link new information to old. Use illustrations, analogies and examples. To explain that a baby grows inside its mother, identify a pregnant woman the child knows or read a picture book featuring a pregnant woman. Say something like, "Billy's mom is about to have a new baby in her family. Have you noticed how big her tummy is? Where do you think the baby might be? The baby is inside Billy's mother—not in her stomach, where the food goes—but in a different place inside the body made just for babies." This explanation ties new information to a common sight for children—a lady with a big tummy.

Children who understand the basics of reproduction sometimes ask, "How can the baby come through a small place like the vagina?" A helpful analogy is to compare the vagina to something children are familiar with. You might say, "What a great question! The vagina is a small opening and a baby's pretty big. Well, the vagina can stretch, like a balloon. You know how you can fill a balloon with air 'til it gets big and round. Then when you let the air out, the balloon goes back down to its normal size. Well, the vagina does the same thing. It can stretch big enough for the baby to pass through, and then go back to its normal size."

In using analogies, be careful not to confuse children further. A very popular children's book tries to explain the concept of orgasm by comparing it to sneezing. I can understand the basis for the analogy—comparing the build-up and release of tension in orgasm to a sneeze. Still, it's easy to imagine a six year old thinking that adults spend a lot of time sneezing when they're making love.

Use simple language and be sure the meanings of new words are clear. When working with young children, less is often more when it comes to helping them begin to understand complex issues. In workshops with primary teachers, I use an activity that asks them to develop simple, concrete explanations for:

- adoption
- childbirth
- clitoris
- erection
- intercourse
- life cycle
- menstruation
- penis
- reproduction
- uterus
- vagina
- disability

First I acknowledge that many of these concepts—such as menstruation, erection and orgasm—are not introduced at the kindergarten level. But, as all teachers know, children often ask questions about things they've seen on TV or heard from older kids. So we need to be prepared to break down ideas appropriately. This activity helps to practice creating the "less" answers to challenging questions.

Next I ask teachers to brainstorm general guidelines for making ideas concrete. Once they have a clear sense of some practical ways to simplify their ideas, I have them get into small groups, each of which I assign two sexual terms. The task is to create no more than three simple sentences that explain their assigned terms in a way that kindergarten or first grade students would understand.

This activity works well because we are forced to identify the least amount of information children need to begin to understand an abstract concept. It helps us get into the child's mind set. What questions or worries might the children have? What basic messages do we want to get across to them?

Let's take menstruation. How far would you go in explaining this to a five year old? Here are three simple sentences that were created in one of my training sessions:

1. Menstruation, or having periods, is something that happens to girls when they get older.
2. It helps make a girl's body able to have babies.
3. It's something natural and healthy that all girls experience.

These are not the only, or even the best, three sentences that could be created to explain menstruation. However, they do cut through the complexities to carve out a very basic message. Notice that sentence 3 lets children know that menstruation is a normal and natural process that happens to all girls. This sentence provides the "music" that goes with the factual information.

Teachers (and parents) vary in how comfortable they feel about answering children's questions. It comes as a relief to many teachers when I tell them they can respectably choose to give a "less" answer to complex questions. As you get more and more comfortable with the topic of sexuality, you will also become more skilled at composing music to play in these brief explanations.

What three sentences would you create for the concept of erection? Many young children have observed a baby boy's erection, perhaps during a diaper change, and they're very curious. Why does the penis stand up? Is it OK? Is it going to go back down? The following three sentences respond to children's typical concerns:

1. Sometimes a boy's or a man's penis gets stiff.
2. It's something that happens to penises from time to time and it's OK.
3. It often means the boy is having a good feeling in his penis.

These sentences assume the child already knows the term penis. (This term can be described with these three sentences: The penis is the body part of a man or boy that hangs between his legs. The penis is very sensitive and usually feels good when it is touched. A boy uses his penis to urinate or "pee" and for sexual intercourse when he's grown up.) The basic message is that "standing" penises are normal. The information that penises are the source of good feelings conveys the music. In simple exchanges like this, adults let children know they're willing to discuss the idea of sexual pleasure.

Remember that this training activity is designed to get adults in the habit of breaking down information, thinking of "less" answers and composing "music" to accompany the facts. In reality, you wouldn't talk to children in the rigid format of the three sentences. You'd probably begin by asking a question or two, then giving information in your own words and in a style that fits the situation.

Practice making ideas concrete by creating sentences for some of the other words on the list. Compare your responses to those presented in Appendix A. Or use the examples as a springboard for your own ideas. Take heart in the fact that by the time most children reach third or fourth grade, they are more capable of understanding fuller explanations.

Chapter 3

Answering Children's Questions: Guidelines, Tips and Suggestions

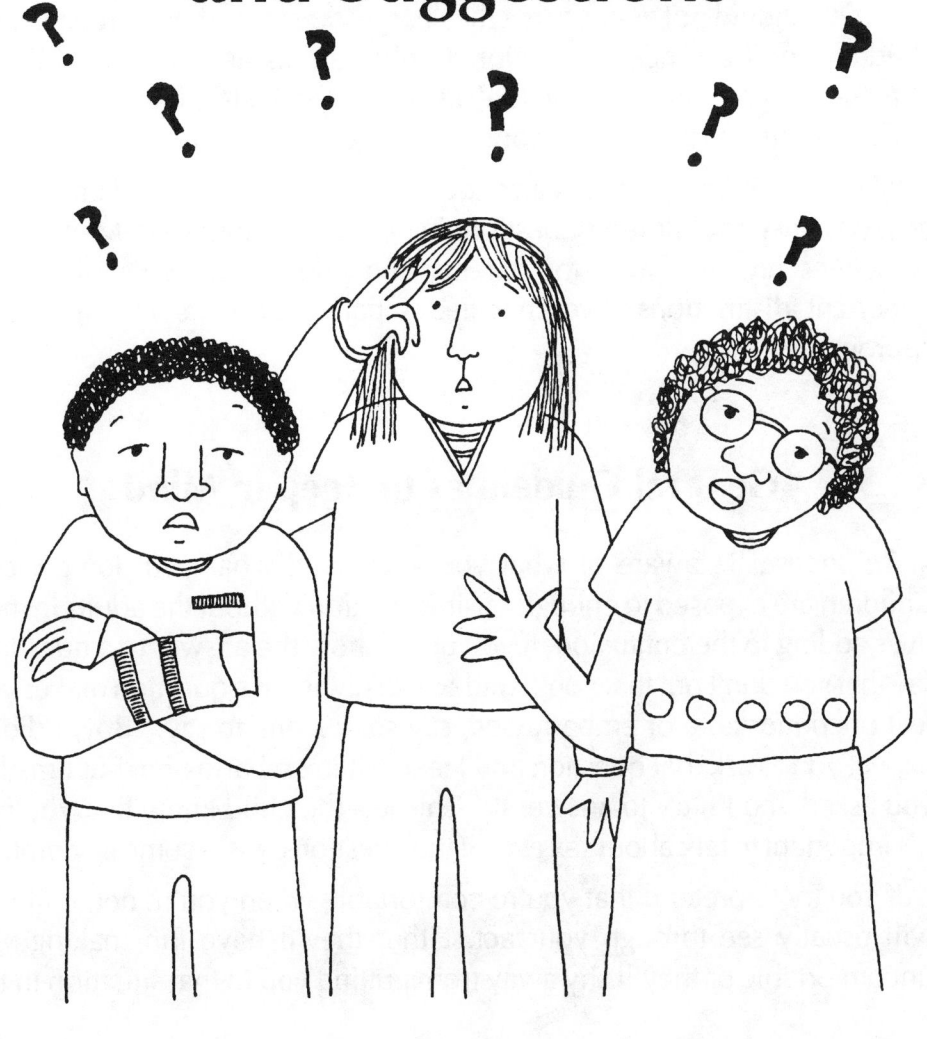

Children vary greatly when it comes to asking questions about sexuality. Some ask freely very often. Others ask only when something perplexes them. Still others never ask. There are many reasons why some children never ask questions:

- They may not have a curious nature.
- They may be shy.
- They may prefer to find their own answers to questions.
- They may have picked up a message from adults around them that it's not OK to ask questions about sexuality.

Parents should not assume that they have done something wrong if their children don't ask questions. Nor should parents assume that children don't need information if they don't ask. Chapter 5 offers ideas for ways to initiate conversations and respond to teachable moments.

Whether you're a parent or an educator, the guidelines listed below will help you answer children's questions in nonthreatening ways. Many of the guidelines are the same for parents and educators. When there are important distinctions, I've specified separate answers that might be appropriate.

General Guidelines to Keep in Mind

Be honest. Be aware of what you know and what you don't know. Children are exposed to enough misinformation without the adults in their lives adding to the confusion. If you don't know the answer to a question, say that you don't but that you'll find out. Likewise, if a question makes you feel uncomfortable or embarrassed, say so. It's fine to say, "Boy, I didn't expect you to ask that question and I feel a little embarrassed, but I'm glad you asked and I'll try to answer it." This lets the child know that you feel it's important to talk about sex even if the question causes some discomfort.

If you try to pretend that you're comfortable when you're not, children will usually see through your act. Either they'll have fun making you uncomfortable or they'll shy away from putting you in that situation in the future. Whatever you do, don't lie to children. This is bad music that causes them to mistrust you in the future.

Answer questions in age-appropriate language. Use simple, concrete answers and words children can understand. When responding to four to six year olds, remember that less is better than more.

Avoid technical language and jargon. When you introduce a new term, make sure you define it or offer an illustration or a colloquial term that children already know. If you're talking about the penis, you might say, "The penis is the part of a boy's body that hangs between his legs. A boy uses his penis to urinate, or pee. Some people call the penis the 'pee pee,' 'privates,' or some other name. The name we'll use here at school (or in this family) is penis."

When talking about HIV/AIDS, avoid technical jargon, such as "sexual contact" or "exchange of body fluids." Although kindergarten students need to understand how difficult it is to get AIDS, there's no reason to inform them of the specific ways that HIV *is* transmitted. But by the time children reach fourth or fifth grade, they need to know that there are three basic ways to get the virus that causes AIDS: (1) by sharing needles to shoot drugs, (2) by having sexual intercourse with someone who has the virus (intercourse refers to sex when the penis is in the vagina, when the penis is in the anus, or when the mouth is used on the vulva or penis); and (3) by passage of the virus from mother to child during pregnancy or childbirth.

Find out more about the child's question. Ask, "What do you think about that?" "How do you think it happens?" or "What have you heard about that?" Make sure your tone sounds accepting and not disapproving. This technique can be helpful to parents and teachers alike. Besides giving you a clearer idea of the child's question, it offers you a couple of extra minutes to figure out what you want to say.

Check out the child's understanding. After you've answered the question, you might ask, "Does that answer your question?" Or have the children tell you what they understood.

Beyond these general guidelines, I'd like to discuss a few types of questions that parents and teachers find particularly challenging.

What About Personal Questions?

When it comes to personal questions, parents and teachers should follow different sets of guidelines. Let's talk about parents first. Naturally, if you are a parent you will make your own decisions about how far to go in answering personal questions from your children. When you share memories about the worries, anxieties, challenges and thrills you experienced while growing up, it can deepen your relationship with your sons and daughters. It gets trickier, though, when children ask about your sexual experiences: How old were you when you had sex the first time? Did you have sex when you were a teenager? Have you ever had sex with anyone other than mom or dad?

How should you respond? Use your own judgment but know that you won't be a "bad" parent if you don't answer these questions. Children are naturally curious, but they should know that some things are private. (They'll appreciate this fact later when they want more privacy themselves.) In fact, some children get overwhelmed by too much knowledge about their parents' sexual behavior. Elementary teachers can attest to this fact because they frequently hear children's worries and concerns about their parents' behavior.

On the other hand, there are parents who've had positive experiences talking openly with their children about some parts of their sexual experience, especially as their children enter adolescence. Another way of handling these questions is to discuss, in general terms, how people make decisions about sex without talking explicitly about your own behavior. You will have to decide how much to share with your child, based on your feelings, the relationship you have with your son or daughter, and your child's personality.

By contrast, teachers have to be more careful about answering personal sexuality questions. Some are harmless: Are you married? Do you have a baby? Did it hurt when you had your baby? What was it like when you had your first wet dream? Teachers will make individual decisions about answering questions like these. Students like to connect with teachers on a human level, to hear about a teacher's feelings in a given situation or to know something about a teacher's life outside of school.

As a teacher, however, you shouldn't answer questions about your personal sex life. Why? First, students who hear about their teachers' sexual behavior have a hard time keeping such "juicy" information confidential. Second, this is just the kind of discussion that some parents and concerned citizens worry about. These parents fear that teachers who are leading very different lives from their own will discuss their personal values and experiences with students.

Children are naturally curious about a teacher who sits down with them and talks openly about sexual issues. By fourth or fifth grade, they are quite likely to ask questions such as, "Do you have sex?" or "Have you ever used a condom?"

Once when I was co-teaching with a man of a different ethnic group than mine, the fifth graders asked if the two of us were having sex together. We told the group that our personal behavior was private, but we explained that two people can talk openly about sex without actually having sex together. Then the students wanted to know what happened when a white man and a black woman had sex. We realized that we were still the object of their fantasies but felt very comfortable answering this general question.

The best response to the question, "How old were you when you had sex the first time?" is, "What I did is personal for me, but we can talk in general. Do you want to know how old most people are when they have sex the first time? There's no set answer here." Go on to talk about the different choices people make rather than your own sexual behavior.

A Question of Values

When children ask what's right or wrong in given situations, they're asking value-laden questions. Parents should answer these questions forthrightly because they're responsible for passing their values on to their children. Of course, it's always best for these discussions to be two-way, parents should make sure they hear what children think about issues, too, especially as their sons and daughters get older.

It's different for teachers because they're educating other people's children. Teachers must *not* impose their personal values in the classroom. If a ten year old asks whether abortion is murder, answer by discussing the range of values held in our society. An educator's task is to help students examine values held by different groups in the community, including their own families. Unless they are teaching in an organization that embraces a clear set of values supported by parent members, teachers should not give an opinion on controversial issues such as abortion or premarital sex, even if the students push to hear what the teacher thinks.

Most school and community programs identify a set of underlying values on which sexuality education is based. Typically, these values are considered to be shared by most members of the community. Rather than preaching, teachers and youth workers use those underlying values to guide the style and content of their communication with students and group members. Such underlying values compose the melody of the music they play in their programs.

Values that are supported in many programs around the country include:

- Children should have access to age-appropriate information about sexuality.
- Parents are the primary sexuality educators of their children. Parents, rather than educators, have the responsibility of transmitting specific values related to sexual behavior. Schools and community agencies should function as partners with parents in providing sexuality education.
- The worth and dignity of all individuals should be recognized; all individuals should be treated with respect, regardless of their gender, race, age, religion, culture or sexual orientation.
- Sexuality is a natural, positive aspect of the human personality.
- It's wrong to exploit or take unfair advantage of others.
- The human body, as well as all of the associated bodily functions, is natural and good.

- It's best for children to postpone initiating sexual intercourse and other risky sexual behaviors beyond the early adolescent years.
- It's best for adolescents to postpone parenthood until they've completed high school and started a career. They can manage this by abstaining from sexual intercourse or by using an effective method of contraception.

Having a set of underlying values guides teachers in answering certain kinds of questions. For example, a fifth grader once asked me, "What happens when a 20-year-old man has sex with a nine-year-old girl?" The value (It's wrong to exploit or take unfair advantage of others.) allows the teacher to take a strong stand here and say that it's definitely wrong for any adult to have sex with a nine-year-old child. (This question and a possible answer are included in this chapter in the sample questions section.)

If you don't know the values that guide your sex education program, consult your principal or agency administrator. You may have to advocate for the development of a list of underlying values.

Examples of Questions and Answers

There's no one right way to respond to children's questions about sexuality. But in my experience teachers and parents have really appreciated hearing specific answers to questions. So I've included some examples of my answers for your consideration.

Preschool through First Grade Questions (ages four to seven)

Where do babies come from?

"Where do you think babies come from? (Briefly discuss the child's beliefs.) Babies grow in a special place inside their mothers' bodies. This place is warm and cozy and made just to hold the baby. This special place is called the uterus."

How does the baby get in the uterus?

"The baby starts from a tiny little egg (Draw a dot with a pencil to show how small.) that is already in the woman's body. But the woman needs help from a man to make a baby. The man has something special in his body, called sperm, that has to join with the egg inside the woman's body. When the sperm joins the egg, the baby starts to grow."

How does the sperm join with the egg?

"Good question. The sperm has to leave the man's body and get inside the woman's body. The sperm leaves the man's body through an opening at the end of his penis. The sperm gets into the woman's body through an opening between her legs called the vagina. So the man puts his penis into the woman's vagina and the sperm goes from his body into her body, where it can meet the egg. Now you tell me how the sperm joins with the egg."

Why don't girls stand up to pee?

"You've noticed that boys stand up and girls sit down when they pee, or urinate. Boys stand up and pee through an opening in their penis. Girls sit down because they pee through an opening between their legs."

Why don't I have a penis (asked by a girl)?

"Boys and girls have many body parts that are the same and some that are different. Boys have a penis. Girls don't have a penis but they have some very special parts that boys don't have. Girls have a vulva—that's what we call the part of a girl's body that is between her legs. (In one-to-one conversations, use "you" language: "your body," "between your legs.") Girls also have a clitoris that is a small part within the vulva. Like the penis in boys, the clitoris is a special part that can bring girls good feelings."

(If the child is still interested, you might go on to say that girls have a part inside their bodies, called the uterus, that can hold a baby if a girl decides to become a mother when she becomes an adult.)

Think about the "musical" messages—the melodies—that come through in these answers:

- The questions were acknowledged as legitimate and answered accordingly.
- The process of reproduction was portrayed as natural yet wondrous.
- Girls' and boys' genitals were described as special and the source of good feelings. The clitoris was specifically named.
- The important role of men in reproduction was acknowledged.
- Parenthood was presented as something optional that a girl can decide about later.

Second and Third Grade Questions (ages seven and eight)

How does the baby get out?

"When the baby is big enough, it comes out through the opening between the mother's legs called the vagina. That's how most babies are born."

(If the child is still interested, you can go on to say, "Some babies are born in a different way. The doctor makes a small opening in the mother's uterus from the outside of her body [point to this part of the body] and takes the baby out that way. Either way the baby is born is fine.")

Does it hurt to have a baby?

"Yes, it usually does hurt when a woman has a baby. But a pregnant woman can learn ways of breathing that make having a baby less painful. And she can have someone else around, like the baby's father, to help make her comfortable. Some women also take medicine to help the pain. Most mothers say that the joy of having a baby makes it easier to deal with the pain."

Why don't boys get breasts?

"Actually, boys do have breasts but their breasts stay pretty flat. When girls become teenagers their breasts get rounder and larger so that they can feed a baby if they decide to have one later on. When boys become men they won't be able to feed a baby from their breasts. But they can take care of a baby by feeding it from a bottle."

How does the baby eat when it's inside its mother?

"The baby does get food when it's in the uterus, but not in the way that you and I eat food with our mouths. The baby is attached to its mother's uterus by a tube called the umbilical cord. Food that the mother eats goes from her body to the baby's body through this cord. This is why it's important for women to eat good, healthy food when they're going to have a baby."

What is sex?

"What do you think sex is?" Depending on the child's answer, you might say, "Sex is a word that can mean a lot of different things. It can mean being a boy or being a girl. For example, someone might ask, 'What is the sex of your baby?' And I would say, 'My baby is a girl.'"

Or you might want to answer by saying, "A lot of people use the word sex to mean sexual intercourse—when a man puts his penis in a woman's vagina. But sex is more than just that. It can include a lot of different ways that two people might touch each other's bodies to show love or to get good feelings."

What is rape?

"Tell me what you've heard about rape." Depending on the response you might say, "Remember when we talked about sex? When adults have sex they might kiss and touch each other's bodies. Sometimes they have intercourse—when the penis goes into the vagina. Sex should only happen when both people want it to happen. Rape happens when one person forces another person to have sex. Rape is not OK. In fact, rape is against the law in our country."

What is a condom?

"What have you heard about condoms?" Depending on the response, you might say, "A condom is something that people can use during sexual intercourse to keep from making a baby or getting certain kinds of diseases (such as AIDS)." This answer will be enough for some children. If not, you can continue by saying, "A condom is something that a man puts on his penis during sex to protect himself or his partner in case either one has a disease. A condom can also allow a man and a woman to have sexual intercourse without making a baby, because it stops the sperm from going into the woman's body to meet an egg."

Here are some of the melodies we are beginning to compose in this round of questions and answers:

- There are many variations in the human experience. Some babies are born vaginally, some via cesarean section. We want children to know that either way of being born is OK.
- The experience of childbirth is not free of pain. We don't want to "whitewash" issues for children, nor do we want to scare them.
- Although men can't experience childbirth or breastfeeding directly, they play an important role in nurturing their children.
- Sex is more than sexual intercourse.
- Sexual behavior should be freely chosen. Forced sex or rape is wrong.
- People have control over their own health. They can protect themselves from sexually transmitted disease and unplanned pregnancy.

Fourth and Fifth Grade Questions (ages nine and ten)

What would you do if your mom and dad separated and your dad got remarried and the stepmother was mean to you?

(If this question gets asked in a group setting, it's best to turn it back to the group. Many children have already had experience with this issue; they'll have ideas and opinions to share.)

"Lots of children worry that they'll end up with a mean stepparent. From a very young age, you've heard fairy tales about wicked stepmothers. That makes it easy for us to think we know all about stepmothers before we ever meet them. We expect them all to be mean and nasty.

Most stepmothers and stepfathers are not mean. But it can be hard for children to get used to having a new 'parent' around. How much will that person tell you what to do? Will she take all of your dad's attention away from you? It's very important for kids to have someone to talk to when they're dealing with this kind of problem. Who are some of the adults you could talk to about a problem like this?"

When a boy gets big, does he have some kind of wet stuff coming out of his penis?

"Yes. As a boy gets older, his body starts to change. His shoulders get wider, hair grows under his arms and his penis gets larger. He begins to produce sperm. His body also makes a fluid that mixes with the sperm before it leaves his body. This fluid is called semen. When the semen comes out of the boy's penis, we say that he's having an ejaculation."

If a penis is in a vagina and the man urinates, what will happen?

"You know that a man urinates through his penis, so it makes sense to wonder whether he might urinate during sexual intercourse. This can't happen. When a man is having intercourse, his body does not let him urinate."

Are tampons better than sanitary napkins?

Parents answering this question are free to communicate their personal preferences. Teachers, as modeled in the answer below, should leave the choice open.

"I don't think either one is better than the other. One advantage to using a tampon, though, is that it allows a girl to go swimming when she's having her period. Both tampons and sanitary napkins are good choices for girls and women. Girls can get advice from their parents about which is best for them to use."

What is a good age to start dating?

A parent can give guidance based on family values. A teacher might say:

"What are your opinions on that?" In the discussion, make the following points: "There's no one right answer here. It's best for you to work this out with your parents. Many young people feel most comfortable going out in groups when they first start to date. Several friends might go to a movie together or to an amusement park. What do you think about that?"

If people don't want you to have sex until you're an adult, why does puberty happen so early in life?

"Boy, that's a great question. It doesn't seem to make much sense for kids to begin puberty so early in life. In the old days, people often married and had children in their teen years. Now things are different.

"But think of it this way. Sex means more than just sexual intercourse. Puberty is a time to learn, to get adjusted to a new body and to figure things out. There's a lot to learn about the kind of man or woman you want to be, about the kind of people you want to be friends with. And there are some ways that young people can be sexual that don't lead to serious consequences. For example, many children discover more about their sexual feelings by touching their own bodies. Some people feel comfortable with this and others don't. It's good to have adults in your life you can talk to about the feelings you're having during puberty."

When a 20-year-old man has sex with a nine-year-old girl, what will happen?

"This is a very important question. If the nine-year-old girl has started having her period, she could get pregnant. If the man has a disease, he could pass it to the girl through sex. But the most important thing here is that a *man,* an adult, is having sex with a *girl.* It is not okay for an adult to have sex with a child. The girl hasn't done anything wrong. She's a child who is being forced or persuaded to have sex by a much older person.

The girl needs to find an adult she can talk to—her mother or father, a school counselor, an aunt or uncle, a neighbor, a teacher. She needs

Answering Children's Questions _____ 45

someone who can help her with this problem. The man needs some help so that he can stop having sex with children. If you know someone in this situation, please encourage your friend to talk to an adult."

How do two women have sex together?

"A lot like the way a man and a woman do. They might kiss and hug, and use their hands and mouths to touch each other's bodies, including the clitoris. The one thing two women can't do is have sexual intercourse where the penis goes into the vagina, because there is no penis."

How many minutes do you have to stay in sexual intercourse? (I love this question. It's a wonderful example of the naivete of children this age who are just trying to figure things out.)

"There's no set amount of time that people have to stay in sexual intercourse. It depends on the two people and how they're feeling at the moment."

☙ ☙ ☙

Before you read the points below, jot down your ideas about the music being played here. Note any questions that you'd answer a little differently. Remember, there's never only one right way to respond to a child's question.

- Stereotypes are harmful, whether we apply them to stepmothers or to any other group. We shouldn't put people in boxes.
- Children's questions about sex and sexual behavior are valid and deserve answers.
- Children should make individual choices about sanitary protection—and other issues—with the help of their parents. It's not up to teachers to recommend one form of protection over another.
- Adults can help children with all kinds of problems and concerns.
- Sex between two women isn't bizarre or unimaginable. Children are naturally curious about what two people of the same sex do because sex is usually described to them as sexual intercourse—penis in vagina.

- Masturbation is a way to discover more about sexual feelings and express such feelings safely during the preadolescent years.
- It's wrong for an adult to have sex with a child. Children in that situation have done nothing wrong; they need adult help.
- Sexual behavior, desires, and interests are very individual matters. There is no one set way to do or feel things.

Chapter 4

Especially for Teachers: Sexuality Education in the Classroom

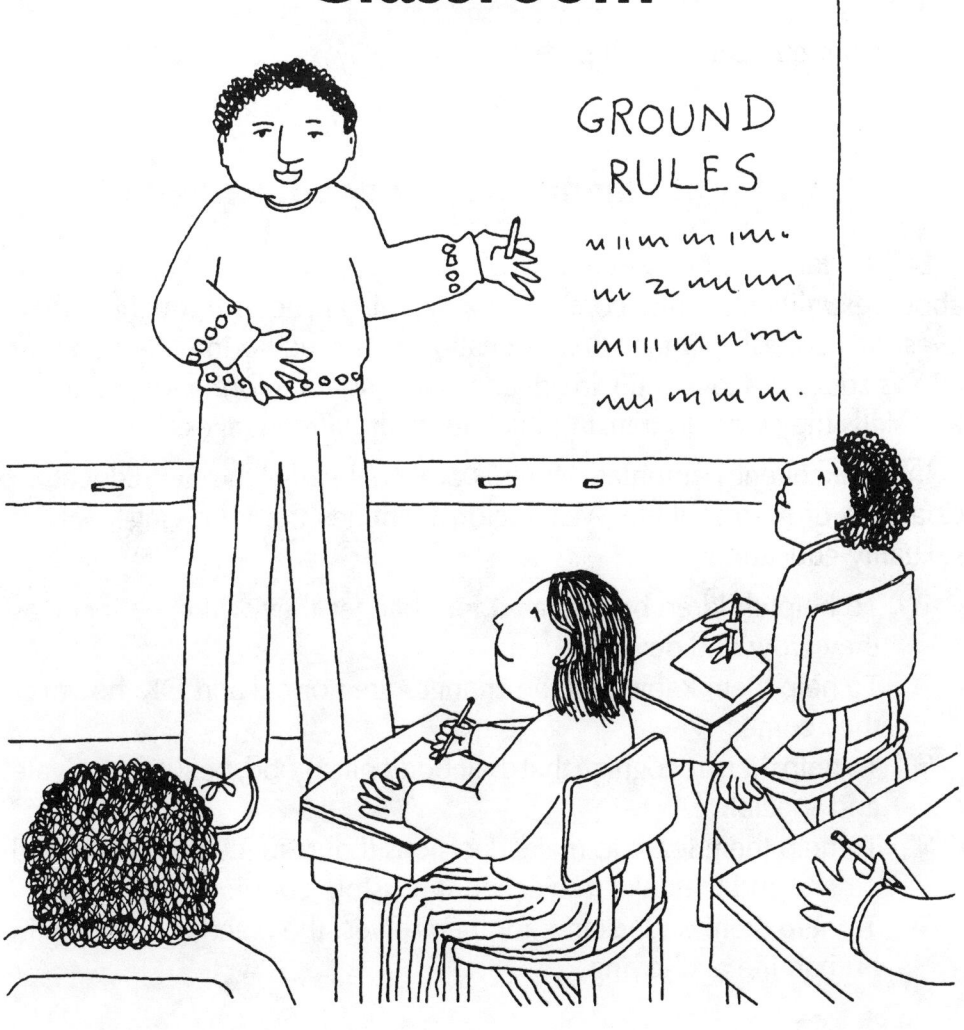

This chapter speaks to teachers about the practice of sexuality education with young children. Whether you are teaching in a school or a community agency, you'll want to explore:
- The goals of planned sexuality education.
- How you feel about teaching sexuality education.
- Teacher training.
- Ways to establish a positive learning climate.
- Handling group discussions.
- Teaching about sexual abuse.
- Male teacher involvement in sexuality education.
- Communicating with parents.

Goals of Planned Sexuality Education

Earlier I talked about the concept of sexual learning—that children learn about sexuality daily and continue that learning process throughout their lives. In contrast, planned sex education is a specific intervention that allows educators to identify in advance the kinds of information, attitudes and skills they want to transmit to children at different ages.

In its excellent pamphlet, *What is Sex Ed Really?* the Sex Education Coalition of Metropolitan Washington identifies the following goals of sexuality education:
- To help children be prepared for changes they will experience as they grow and develop.
- To help them know that the changes are normal and OK, however they come.
- To help them recognize that their bodies are good, beautiful, private and special.
- To help them learn to make decisions that respect themselves and others, and that take into account possible consequences.
- To help them understand, for themselves, the place of sexuality in human life and loving.

Effective sexuality education must be age-appropriate. Parents and teachers who oppose sex education—and they are in the minority—often do so because they have misconceptions about recommended content at various grade levels. For example, teachers in a school district I work with mistakenly thought they'd have to demonstrate contraceptives to elementary school children. They were relieved when they got to review the actual curriculum.

Most curricula for the primary grades deal with the following topics:

- Identifying roles and responsibilities of families.
- Understanding and managing feelings.
- Understanding similarities and differences between boys and girls.
- Understanding basic concepts of reproduction.
- Understanding basic concepts of human growth and development.
- Increasing awareness and appreciation of differences among human beings: their appearance, their family structures, their physical development, their abilities, their feelings in different situations.
- Preventing sexual abuse.
- Identifying people and places who can help with problems.

By the upper elementary years, programs typically deal with topics such as:

- Helping children understand and cope with changes in the family.
- Increasing children's knowledge of the physical, emotional and social changes that accompany puberty.
- Increasing students' social skills—listening, starting conversations, making decisions and being assertive.
- Increasing children's awareness and understanding of themselves.
- Having students explore their feelings and attitudes about peer relationships.
- Increasing preadolescents' motivation and skills to postpone initiation of sexual intercourse.
- Increasing children's comfort with the topic of sexuality.
- Dispelling myths about sexuality and about AIDS.

Especially for Teachers

- Increasing children's acceptance of differences in values, life styles, customs and beliefs in their community.
- Increasing awareness of and skills for preventing or getting help with sexual abuse.

Programs vary greatly in their content. Some variation is needed to tailor individual programs to the specific needs of your community and its families. For instance, a progressive school district in a "high risk" urban area quite appropriately deals with issues of adolescent pregnancy, contraception and sexually transmitted disease with sixth graders. Other school districts postpone the presentation of these topics for a few years because they haven't observed the need for or interest in these topics among their elementary school students. It is always advisable, however, to give teachers the freedom to answer *all* questions (other than personal) that come up in the classroom. The freedom to ask and get age-appropriate answers insures that children will receive the specific information they need in a timely fashion.

Special Concerns About Teaching Sexuality to Young Children

At the beginning of teacher training workshops, I always ask teachers to imagine that they're in their classrooms starting their first sex ed lesson. How do they feel? What are they worried about?

Here's a typical list of their concerns:

- Will children ask embarrassing questions that I can't answer?
- Will I feel comfortable saying sexual words?
- Will the students take the information seriously?
- How far should I go in answering questions?
- Will parents get upset about the lessons?
- Will I be able to pull this off?
- I'm nervous about dealing with child sexual abuse. Will children come to me with stories about being abused? How should I respond?

❦ (From a male teacher) Will the girls feel comfortable talking to me about puberty and menstruation?

These are all valid concerns that must be addressed before teachers feel comfortable taking on the task of sex education. The teachers in the school district I mentioned at the beginning of this chapter are lucky; they get two graduate courses to prepare them for teaching family life education. Without intensive training, most teachers either do an inadequate job or avoid sexuality education altogether.

Training Teachers to Be Prepared

What should be covered in teacher training? Ideally, educators would first deal with their own sexuality by revisiting their upbringing and sorting out their values about a range of sexual topics. It's critical that educators be able to talk about sexual values without imposing their own. This takes practice!

The next level of individual preparation deals with knowledge. Teachers need to have basic information about anatomy, physiology, sexual development, puberty, sexually transmitted diseases and contraception. It would be unreasonable to expect educators to be sexuality experts, but they do have to know the basics. And they need to be aware of what they *don't* know and where they can go for additional information.

Another component of teacher training is skill building. Even though some prospective sexuality educators are certified teachers, they may not be skilled in group facilitation or affective learning techniques. Most sexuality education programs use a small-group format that requires a skilled facilitator to manage the process. Facilitators work at stimulating discussion by encouraging two-way communication with group members, asking open-ended questions and conducting activities that encourage children to learn experientially.

Teachers also need to learn how to use sexual language appropriately, answer children's sexuality-related questions effectively and break down abstract concepts for very young children.

For most teachers, participating in comprehensive training—exploring their own values, gaining relevant knowledge, learning and practicing methods of answering children's sexual questions—increases their comfort with the whole process. By the end of training most of them are still a little nervous but they feel more prepared for the task at hand. Once a teacher actually implements the program at least once, these natural jitters decrease. The more times sexuality educators teach, the more comfortable they become.

I firmly believe that training is even more important than curriculum development. You can give the best curriculum in the country to unprepared teachers and they'll almost surely have a bad experience. The teacher or program leader is the most important variable in determining a program's success.

An effective sexuality educator should:

- Have participated in comprehensive sexuality training.
- Be tolerant or accepting of differing values and points of view.
- Support the underlying values and principles of the program.
- Be well informed about sexual topics.
- Convey warmth and a sense of humor.
- Have explored his or her own attitudes about a variety of sexual issues.
- Feel enthusiastic about teaching sexuality education to young children.
- Have good communication and group facilitation skills.
- Use sexual terminology correctly and comfortably.
- Be familiar with the needs and sensitivities of children who come from various ethnic and socioeconomic backgrounds.

Creating a Positive Learning Environment

An essential step in effective sexuality education is to create an environment in which children feel comfortable, safe and motivated to participate. You can do this in two ways: by conducting some warm-up activities to set the tone, and by beginning to play your music, listening carefully to children, accepting their initial "giggles and wiggles," answering their questions honestly, and talking about yourself as a person in appropriate ways.

Warm-up Activities

Most sexuality programs begin with an activity designed to foster a good climate for learning. Warm-up activities ought to be easy for everyone to get involved in and be related in some way to the content of the program. At their best, these activities break the ice, decrease tension, help children get to know one another (if they don't already), and increase energy for the upcoming program. Children find out through experience that they'll have fun while they learn.

There are a few types of warm-ups that are used over and over in sexuality education. The Name Game asks students to introduce themselves by giving their first names and a positive adjective that begins with the first letter of their name. For example, "I'm Popular Pam." The fun comes when each new person has to introduce everyone who has spoken before. There are also scavenger hunts where children have to find someone who is an only child, has a mother who works outside of the home, has a new baby in the family and so on. Physical activities such as adaptations of musical chairs are also good for creating energy.

Ground Rules

Equally important in setting the tone is the establishment of ground rules. Ground rules help children behave in ways that are respectful of one another and feel safe enough to express their honest feelings or ask what they're afraid may be a silly question. Some teachers get students to create their own ground rules by telling a story that goes something like this:

On the first day of the sexuality education program, Maria asks, "Can a man have a baby?" All of her classmates fall out of their chairs laughing. Maria sits with her head on her desk for the remainder of class. What rules could have been made to keep this kind of thing from happening?

Recommended ground rules include:

- No put downs or teasing.
- Pay attention to other people's feelings.
- No one should ask personal questions or talk about personal matters like parents' behavior or friends' behavior.
- There are no "dumb" questions. You can ask anything you want.
- People have the right not to answer any question they don't want to answer.
- No talking about other students' comments outside of the classroom. Talk in general terms, and never use a student's name when you talk about classroom discussions.
- If you don't feel comfortable talking about a topic in this program, you can pass.

Organized Chaos

Some teachers who are new to sexuality education are surprised by the recommended format. The sessions are supposed to be lively. Students must be actively involved. Discussion should develop spontaneously. If all happens as it's supposed to, sex ed classes are bound to be noisy. Students sometimes buzz with side conversations—not because they are bored—but because they're fully engaged in the topic and can't wait to make their comments heard publicly.

You'll be playing bad music if you spend the bulk of your time on discipline. If children seem particularly unruly during the sessions, you may need to revise your expectations of appropriate behavior or revisit the ground rules by encouraging group members to suggest ways of dealing with the problem behaviors so that the group can work effectively. So you might say, "Everyone is so excited that you're all talking at once and we can't hear each other. What do you think we should do so that we all have a chance to speak and to hear what each person is saying?"

Giggling

Educators often ask me, "Will my students take the program seriously enough?" I think some of us have a need to keep discussions of sexuality somewhat serious because we don't want to be accused of treating the subject frivolously. But experienced teachers know that telling students they're expected to act very mature and not to be silly can set a very restrictive tone.

Let's think about why children giggle. Why do adults giggle? It's often a vehicle for releasing nervousness or discomfort. When we tell children not to giggle, we inhibit their natural behavior, causing them to censor what they say and do. This is very bad music. Most of the giggling takes place at the start of the program. It may be the first time children have had this kind of discussion in school. They may have picked up the idea that sex is a taboo topic and not be sure how to behave. You can help them understand their feelings by explaining the purpose of giggling. Give them a couple of minutes to get all the giggling out. Giggle along with them if you feel like it. Most teachers find that this natural behavior decreases with time.

Truly Silly Questions

We have our groundrule stating that no questions will be viewed as silly, but let's face it, occasionally a kid will ask something just for fun or to get a laugh. "How much weight can an erect penis hold?" is one example. Sometimes its best just to respond lightly, perhaps by saying, "Not much" with a smile and going on to the next question. Have some fun with it but don't reinforce attention-seeking behavior.

Handling Group Discussions: The Question Box

Many sexuality education programs use a helpful technique called the question box. Students are given an opportunity to write their questions anonymously rather than stating them aloud in the group. All you need is a shoe box and a stack of index cards. The question box works best if you pass out index cards and ask all students to write down a question they have about sexuality. Ask students who don't have a specific question to write "no question" on their cards. Then walk around the room and have students place their questions directly in the box. Never have them pass their cards down a row of seats.

You may choose to announce the question box at the beginning of the program, then provide regular opportunities for students to write questions. One advantage of this technique is that you collect the cards at one session and answer them at the next. This gives you time to review the questions and think about the best way to answer them. Since students need to be able to write to participate in this activity, most programs don't introduce the question box until grade three or four.

Here are some hints to help you respond to anonymous questions:

Read each question just as it appears on the index card. If a slang term was used, restate the question using the correct terminology. Suppose a fifth grader asks, "What determines how big a boy's dick gets?" You could say, "'Dick' is a slang term for 'penis'" and then go on with your answer, using the word penis.

Turn "feeling" or value-laden questions back to the group to find out what the children think. An example of a "feeling" question is, "What should you do if you plan to go somewhere with one friend and then someone you like better asks you to do something?"

Encouraging children to answer these questions themselves gives them a chance to reflect on issues and to hear different opinions held by others in the group. "Feeling" questions related to sexual behavior, such as, "How does it feel to make love?" are best answered by you as the adult leader.

Since these questions are supposed to be anonymous, avoid answering

in the second person. A fifth grader once put the following question in the box:

> "This is sort of about menstruation. I have a rash in and on my vagina that I think I got from wearing wet bathing suits over and over again at camp last summer. My mom told me that she had her period when she was 11-1/2 and that girls usually have their periods about the same age their mothers did. I'm now 12 years old and I haven't had my period. Do you think this rash is holding back my period?"

Suppose the leader gives this answer:

> "I'm so glad you wrote this question. First of all, it's perfectly normal that you haven't had your period yet. Some girls get their periods about the same age as their mothers and others don't. Some girls start their periods as young as age nine, others not until age 16. Any of those ages is perfectly normal.
>
> "Even though it's not related to your period, I'm concerned that you've had a rash on your vagina for so long. It's probably something that can be taken care of easily, but you really should get your parents to take you to the doctor to check it out. Any time you notice a rash, a sore or anything unusual on your genitals, it's best to see a doctor and have it checked out."

On the surface, this answer seems good. The leader has discussed normal variations in development and encouraged the girl to see a health practitioner about the rash. But try to imagine how the girl who wrote the question is feeling. It's very possible that she began to squirm as soon as the teacher said, "It's perfectly normal that you haven't had your period yet." And if the girl didn't squirm then, she surely scooted down in her seat when the teacher said, "I'm concerned that you've had a rash on your vagina for so long."

The teacher's use of the pronoun "you" was likely to make the girl feel that her question was no longer confidential. Instead of talking to the whole group, the teacher seems to be talking directly to her.

Especially for Teachers

The following answer is less likely to make the questioner feel as though she's sitting in the spotlight:

> "This is a very important question. Many girls worry when they haven't gotten their periods by a certain age. It's true that some girls start their periods about the same age as their mothers, but many don't. Some begin a lot earlier and some a lot later than their mothers. It's perfectly normal for a girl to begin her period as early as age nine or as late as 16, even if her mother started at 12. It makes sense to think that something like a rash could be holding back a girl's period, but that's not at all likely.
>
> "Still, anytime a person has a rash on the vagina, the penis or even on the face, it's a worry. So it's always best to go to a doctor or a clinic to check things out and just make sure everything is OK. It's good for all of you to tell your parents or some other adult, maybe the school nurse, whenever you notice anything unusual about your body."

This answer isn't very different from the first in tone, but it uses the third person ("many girls," "a person"), thereby keeping the discussion focused on the entire group. That's so even in the one case where the second person is used ("all of you"). The question box activity promises children anonymity, so be careful to keep the discussion safe.

When you get a vague question in the question box, all you can do is make your own interpretation and answer accordingly. An example of a vague question is, "If several boys do it to one girl, what happens?"

A leader might respond:

> "I'm going to assume that 'do it' means to have sexual intercourse. This is a very serious question. What happens? Well, many things could happen. First, if the girl has started having periods, she could get pregnant. Second, if any of the boys has a disease, she could get the disease. Since the girl had intercourse with more than one person, she has more of a chance of getting a disease. I wonder how old these

children are. Did they know enough to do things to prevent pregnancy or disease?

"The last—but most important—thing that could happen has to do with feelings. How did the girl feel about what happened? Did she want to have sex with several boys or did they force her? How did the boys feel? Were any of them pressured by their friends to do this? If the girl or any of the boys felt pressured to have sex, it was probably a bad experience for them. Remember, it's wrong to force people to do things they don't want to do."

"What happens" questions tend to be vague. Here the leader assumed the student was asking what happens when a group of boys have sex with a girl. But the question might mean what happens if a girl has sex with several boys over the same period of time, a month or so. Don't try to cover all bases. If you haven't made the right interpretation, students can—and usually do—put another question in the box. I often respond to "what happens" questions about sexual behavior by discussing three issues: pregnancy, disease and feelings.

Answer explicit questions honestly, but avoid giving sex instruction. If children know enough to ask a question, they deserve an age-appropriate answer. If responsible adults don't answer children's questions, we leave sexuality education in the hands of peers and the media.

Preadolescents often ask questions like, "What's a blow job?" or "How do homosexuals have sex?" Sometimes when children ask these questions, they already know the answer. They may be testing you to see what you will say. Other times they are truly perplexed. How can you explain a blow job without giving sex instruction? You could say: "'Blow job' is a slang term. It usually means using the mouth on the penis during sex."

Notice that I chose the words "using the mouth on the penis" rather than "sucking or licking the penis during sex." I find that words like "suck" and "lick" evoke visual images I'm not intending to elicit. It's best to answer explicit questions briefly, in an honest but matter-of-fact manner.

Use inclusive language. Avoid being sexist. Use "he or she" to refer to

Especially for Teachers

doctors, or use "she" half of the time. Replace words in your vocabulary that end in "man" such as chairman (chair), policeman (police officer) and fireman (fire fighter).

Be careful, too, to avoid "heterosexist" terms. Heterosexism refers to the belief that all people are or should be heterosexual. I once heard a program leader explain a blow job by saying, "It's when a woman performs oral sex on a man." First of all, some young people don't know what oral sex is. But more importantly, women are not the only people who might perform a blow job.

With a little thought, it's easy to answer questions without referring to gender. Use words like "partner" rather than boyfriend, girlfriend, husband or wife. When talking about romance and love, choose words that convey the idea that romance occurs between members of the same sex as well as members of the opposite sex. Most people need to retrain themselves to give up heterosexism, but it's the only way to make sexuality discussions relevant to all children—including those who grow up to realize they're gay or lesbian.

Teaching About Sexual Abuse

Sexual abuse is one of the most difficult topics for adults to explain to children. We don't want to scare them. But we do want them to be aware of the problem, to develop skills that can help them get away from potentially dangerous situations and to know how to get help if something like this happens to them. Our goal is to increase children's ability to avoid abuse without giving them the idea that they are completely responsible for keeping themselves safe. How can we expect five to ten year olds to assume that kind of responsibility?

I've become increasingly concerned about the "good touch/bad touch" approach to teaching about sexual abuse. We tell children that there are two kinds of touch—good and bad—and that bad touching occurs when they are touched on the sexual parts of their bodies: the vulva, breasts, penis or buttocks. Because young children are concrete thinkers, they interpret what we're saying to mean that *any* touch on the sexual parts of the body is bad touching. This is horrible music.

In one school district that recommends the good touch/bad touch approach, elementary teachers are noticing that their primary students say things like, "Ruby (a classmate) 'bad touched' me." And older students ask, "Suppose somebody 'bad touches' you and you like it?" We have to do a better job of differentiating between the playful touch of another child (who has equal power) and the abusive touch of an older person. Of course children still need protection from classmates of the same age who are bigger and stronger than they are.

Most importantly, we need to let children know that some touches on the sexual parts of the body are desirable and enjoyable. When they grow up they will probably want those touches from some special person(s). Even when touch is not desired it can feel good and this is also confusing for young children.

So how do we respond to this dilemma? I recommend that we eliminate the simplistic concept of good and bad touching and begin to teach children a more complex set of ideas. In my workshops, I present four basic clues that we can give children to help them recognize a potentially abusive situation:

1. Someone wants to look at or touch the sexual parts of their bodies for no good reason. Examples of good reasons include a doctor giving a physical, a parent bathing a young child, a parent checking out an injury, a friend patting them on the buttocks after a good play during a game.
2. An older more powerful person—typically a teenager or an adult—tries to get them to do something that they don't really want to do. In some cases a child of the same age can be bigger, stronger and, therefore, intimidating. The important thing here is to clarify the power difference in an abusive situation.
3. They sense that there is something strange about the situation. It just doesn't feel comfortable or they get a queasy (uh-oh) feeling inside.

Especially for Teachers

Whenever children feel that a situation just isn't right, they should talk to an adult about it.
4. The adult or teenager in the situation asks or tells them to keep their behavior secret. Or maybe they just sense that the behavior would not take place if another adult was around.

These four clues can help children to use their heads to figure out if something inappropriate is happening. If children become aware of even one of these warning signals, they should find an adult to help them. We must let girls and boys know that there are some things they can do to help prevent or deal with sexual abuse but that they are not bad or irresponsible if they don't do these things. Children cannot be held accountable for keeping themselves safe. That job is up to us as adults.

When the Teacher Is a Man

Male teachers express concern about the issue of sexual abuse. In fact, some have been told by their administrators that they should never touch a student for any reason. This is unfortunate because there are some students who would not get a caring touch during the day if they didn't get it from their teacher.

Men need to be involved in sexuality education at every level, but especially with this age group. If men are comfortable teaching about sexuality, students tend to be comfortable. Young children who have positive experiences talking openly with men about sex learn life-long lessons. Girls learn that sex can be discussed freely with members of the other sex. Boys get to observe an adult role model who is sensitive, nonjudgmental and caring.

In the preadolescent years, though, both girls and boys need some separate sessions with other children and an adult of their same sex. Girls seem less comfortable asking all of their questions about menstruation and sanitary protection when boys are in the room. Boys are less likely to ask about spontaneous erections or masturbation when girls are in the room.

For this reason some school districts conduct one or two separate sessions that they call "personal concerns" sessions. The sessions are introduced as a time for boys and girls to freely ask their personal questions, rather than a time when they will receive information that should be kept private from the other sex. The personal concerns sessions can be facilitated by male and female teachers, counselors, educators from an outside agency or administrators.

Teachers Learning About Parents

When I began my work as a sexuality educator I had a rather warped view of parents. Because I spent most of my time interacting with children and adolescents, I could only see family communication patterns through their eyes. Therefore, I tended to blame parents for much of their children's confusion about sexuality.

After about five years in the field, I joined the staff at a company called Mathtech to work on a major national project designed to help parents become more effective sexuality educators. When I realized that I would be conducting workshops with parents, I got very nervous. Would they question my expertise? Would they resist new knowledge and perspectives? Would they have a problem with their children learning more about their sexuality? I was sure the answer to all those questions would be "yes."

In the true spirit of the self-fulfilling prophecy, I had a lot of difficulty in my first parent groups. I thought poorly of parents and I doubted my own expertise. Parents perceived this immediately and responded accordingly. As time went by and I heard more from parents about their confusing childhood experiences, daily challenges, concern about what was best for their children and desire to do what was best, my attitude changed considerably. Also, my success with the programs increased dramatically.

I no longer have an "us" versus "them" attitude motivating me to want to "whip parents into shape." Today, I get very uneasy when I see parents depicted in stereotyped, incompetent ways in the media and even in our own sexuality education films. It is my heartfelt belief that educators must work as partners with parents in the delivery of sexuality education to children.

If you are an educator who views parents as a part of the problem rather than a part of the solution, please take note. Sometimes we helpers—teachers, social workers, youth workers, counselors, health professionals—have the most contact with particularly troubled families and allow these experiences to color our view of all parents. Find some opportunities to interact with a range of parents from a variety of backgrounds. Listen to them and learn from them. You'll find that most parents are doing the best that they can given the knowledge, understanding and awareness they currently possess.

Parents and Teachers as Partners Providing Sexuality Education

Parents, too, need to hear the right music from sexuality educators. Whenever you conduct a program with young children, inform parents ahead of time about the specific content, aims and underlying values of the program. By involving them from the start, you communicate the value that your school or agency wants to be their partner in the provision of sexuality education. Your goals should include giving parents a say in the kind of sexuality-related information their children will receive, and suggesting ways that parents can communicate about sexuality with their sons and daughters at home.

Here are some strategies for achieving these goals:

1. Involve parents as members of an ongoing advisory committee that reviews program content and approves all print and audiovisual resources.
2. Invite parents to a meeting so they can find out more about the program and view a sampling of the films you plan to use.
3. Give parents the opportunity to "opt their children out" of the

program. There are some people who, for religious or personal reasons, prefer not to have their children participate in discussions of sexuality outside their homes. We must respect these parents' beliefs.

4. Assign homework that children can complete with their parents. Homework activities can balance the roles of home and school by supporting the parents as primary sex educators of their children. Through joint homework activities, parents gain opportunities to influence their children's developing values. The simple act of doing homework together results in increased family communication about sexuality. And if the homework assignment is designed the right way, that communication will involve active listening and opinion sharing on both sides.

5. At the end of the program, send home an evaluation form designed to get parents' input about the effectiveness of the program.

6. Offer programs directly to parents to help them become more effective sex educators. In some communities such programs are offered by school counselors, social workers or community educators rather than teachers. Parents of young children often worry about handling children's questions about sex and about dealing with everyday incidents at home (sex play, use of slang terms, masturbation).

   Depending on the amount of parental involvement in your school or agency, this can be a wonderful option. It's also helpful to offer joint sessions for parents and preadolescents. Some mothers and fathers jump at the chance to come to a sexuality program with their children at a critical point in their children's sexual development.

Chapter 5

Especially for Parents: Sexuality Education at Home

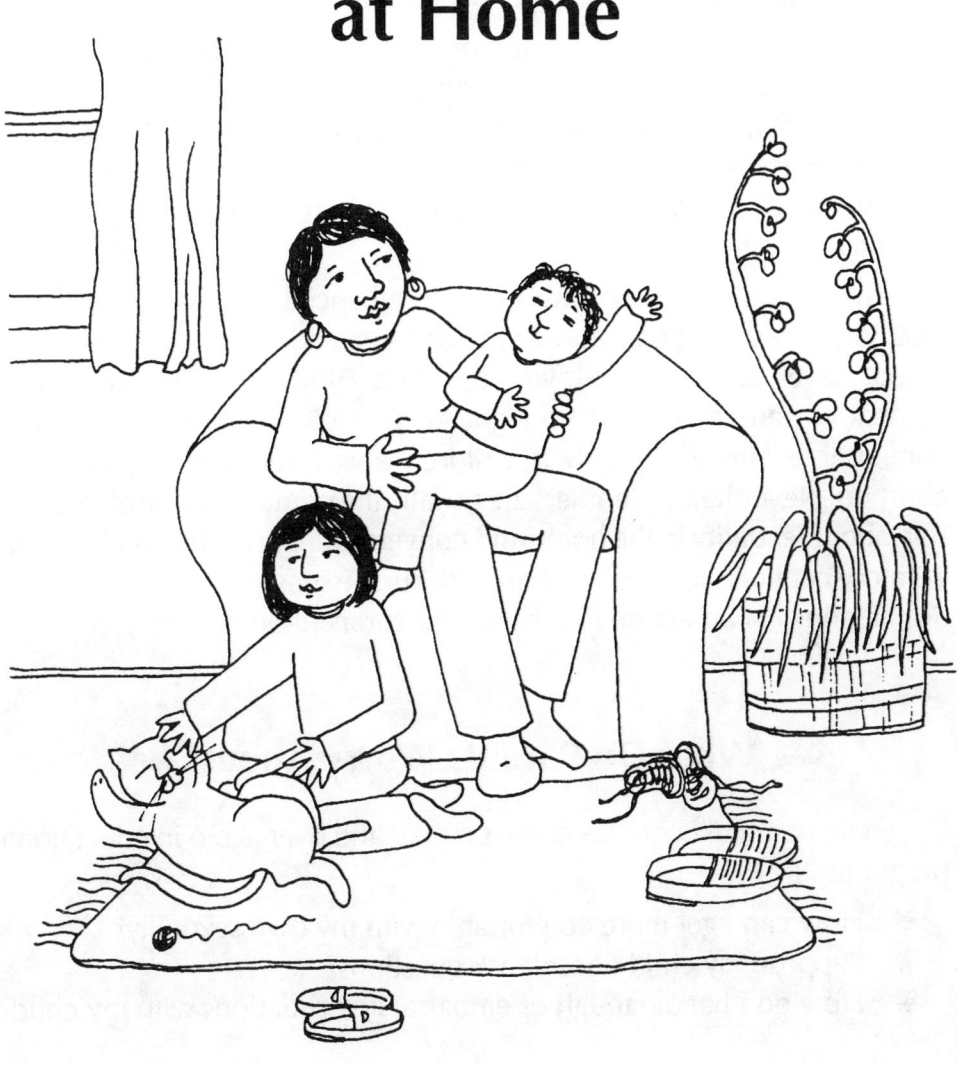

Today's parents face a challenging task in trying to be the primary sexuality educators of their children. Your children are exposed to much more explicit sexuality information from society than you or I ever were. It's virtually impossible for you to limit what your sons and daughters learn on a daily basis. You might be feeling uncertain about what to tell your children in the 1990s. During my workshops, parents have made comments such as, "I know what I believe but I don't want to push my old fashioned values on my children," or, "I don't know what I can tell my child about healthy sexuality given the AIDS situation."

Most of you are juggling...your work, child rearing, your own relationships. Some of you might also be struggling to put food in your family's mouths, to keep a roof over your heads, or perhaps to manage a personal problem with drugs, alcohol, unemployment or violence. Understandably, sexuality education is one small, albeit important, part of your busy agendas.

I have found that most parents, from all social and economic backgrounds, care very deeply about their children and want to influence their sexual development in positive ways. In a 1988 Harris Poll almost 60 percent of parents of seven to eighteen year olds reported feeling very comfortable talking with their children about sex, birth control and abortion. Nevertheless, mothers are usually the primary source of information about sexuality in the home and conversations are more likely to deal with conception and puberty than with such issues as petting, masturbation, feelings of attraction to others, or contraception.

What Do Parents Worry About?

Certain parental concerns come up over and over again in educational programs:
- How can I get more comfortable with my own sexuality?
- Suppose my child doesn't ask questions?
- How do I handle tough or embarrassing situations with my child?

- How should I respond to advanced sexuality questions from young children?

How Can I Get More Comfortable with My Own Sexuality?

Most of us have grown up in homes and a society that give ambivalent messages about sex. "Do it, Do it, Do it!....Sex is dirty; save it for the one you love....It feels good....Men should; women shouldn't....Sex is best when it is spontaneous....Wait until you're married...." What messages did you hear when you were growing up? What were you taught about your own body? What names were you given for the sexual parts? How comfortable were your parents or other caretakers with the topic? What was their basic message about sex? What did they tell you about being a boy or a girl? What did they show and tell you about being affectionate, relating to others, showing love, feeling sexual pleasure and being responsible?

If you've never thought about these questions, take a few minutes now. Discuss them with your partner, a friend or perhaps a parent. The messages you learned about sexuality as a child are still influencing you in a variety of ways. For example, you may find that you rely on your parents' model of sex education. Or possibly you were so turned off by your parents' approach, that you've gone to the opposite extreme. Which of their messages do you agree with today? With which do you now disagree? Why? How do you want your son's or daughter's sexuality education to compare with your own?

Many parents report that the more they talk about their own feelings and values, the more comfortable they become with the topic of sexuality. Spend some time reviewing the books listed in Appendix C and choose a couple for your personal library. Many of us have reached adulthood with little or no information about sexuality and will remain uninformed unless we actively seek out new knowledge. You'll probably find that you feel even more comfortable with the subject once you've learned or relearned some of the basic facts and know where to find answers to any other questions.

Finally, explore your community—schools, health centers, youth-serving organizations, social service agencies, Planned Parenthoods, churches or synagogues—to find a sexuality education program for parents. Many of these organizations provide such programs on an ongoing or as-needed basis. You also may find a program that you can attend *with* your preadolescent son or daughter. Most parents who have managed to participate in these programs say that it was well worth the time and energy. In fact some of them ask for additional sessions at the end of the program or come back for reunions six months later.

Suppose My Child Doesn't Ask Questions?

Children come into this world with their own personalities. You have surely noticed this if you have more than one child. The human personality can be influenced by life experiences but there seems to be a basic core, a basic style that is each child's natural preference. What have you noticed about your own children? Does your daughter ask questions about everything? Or is she more likely to mull ideas over by herself?

I know experienced sex educators who have been very frustrated by a son or daughter who doesn't ask questions or engage much in conversations about sexuality. On the other hand some of my colleagues have kids who thrive so much on the open communication in their homes that they become the junior sexuality educators of their peer groups.

Each child is unique. If your son or daughter doesn't ask questions, bring the subject up yourself in natural ways. Try not to make a big deal out of it. Share a thought about a TV show or news story. Allow your younger children to overhear your conversations with their older siblings, when appropriate. Share your own feelings and keep your sense of humor working. In several projects I've worked on, we asked preadolescents why they avoided conversations about sexuality with their parents.

They listed the following complaints:
- They act like teachers.
- They get too serious.

- They take too long to explain something.
- They pick the wrong time to bring it up.
- They don't laugh enough.
- They don't talk about feelings.

Some parents have found success bringing up the subject of sex during a car ride. In those situations you typically have time to spare and your child is a captive audience. Also, the discussion may not feel as intense in the car because there is no way to maintain real eye contact.

Whatever you do, don't take your child's apparent lack of interest as a signal to leave the topic of sexuality alone. Research conducted by Columbia University professor Fritz Ianni in ten diverse U.S. communities revealed that adolescents reflected the values of their parents, neighborhoods and ethnic groups much more than any "youth culture." So your role in shaping your children's values is just as powerful now as in past generations.

Remember, children who are introverted often take in more from a conversation than the talkers. You might be happily surprised to discover that your more quiet child talks with friends about ideas that you thought had fallen on deaf ears.

How Do I Handle the Tough Situations?

Think about how comfortable you would be dealing with the following situations. Rate yourself on a scale from 1 to 5 depending on your comfort level for each question (1=very uncomfortable, 5=very comfortable).

1. How would you feel explaining intercourse to your child?
2. How would you feel if you discovered your child masturbating?
3. How would you feel describing the birth process to your child, including delivery and how the baby comes out of the woman?
4. How comfortable would you be if your child saw you nude?
5. How would you feel describing the menstrual cycle to your son? Wet dreams?
6. How would you feel describing the menstrual cycle to your daughter? Wet dreams?

7. How do you feel when hugging, kissing, and showing affection to your partner when your children are present?
8. How would you feel if you discovered your five-year-old daughter playing doctor with the five-year-old neighbor boy?
9. How would you feel if your child walked in on you and a partner having sex?

For most parents, these are uncomfortable situations. Even parents who are professional sexuality educators confess that it is much harder to be "cool" when dealing with their own sons or daughters. These are typical situations that occur in most homes. So what do you do?

Let's take as an example number 2 above. If you discover your child masturbating or involved in sex play, you need to ask yourself several questions:

- Why is she doing that? What meaning does it have for her?
- What message do I want to give?
- What should I do?

Obviously, you'll need to take some deep breaths, talk to yourself for a minute, and then respond. Let's take the situation of walking in on your five-year-old daughter playing doctor with a five-year-old boy from the neighborhood. Ask yourself the first question: Why are they exploring each other's bodies? Reassure yourself that these five year olds are not "having sex" together in a adult sense. They are probably curious about each other's bodies or might be mimicking behavior they've seen at home or on TV.

What message do you want to give? Possibly you want your daughter to know that her body is private and that she should not let other people look or touch unless she wants them to. Maybe you want her to know that boys and girls have different body parts and that it is normal for her to be curious.

What should you do? What message would you give your daughter if you:

- Ignore the behavior.
- Reprimand both children and send the friend home?

74 ———————————————————————— *When Sex Is the Subject*

- Create a "teachable moment" by using the opportunity to tell the children about sexual anatomy.
- Distract the children with another activity.
- Send the friend home and discuss body differences and appropriate play with your daughter.
- Calmly tell the children that their bodies are private and that they should keep their clothes on when they play together.

There are no clear right or wrong answers here, but it's helpful to examine the attitudinal message inherent in each response. Your individual values and comfort level will dictate the specific messages you wish to communicate in your family. What's important is that you pay attention not only to your words but to the music that you play when you respond to a situation. Are you communicating the idea that the human body is good and natural or nasty and unmentionable? Are you presenting yourself as a resource for sorting out a concern or worry, or someone to avoid when the subject is sex? Are you satisfying their curiosity or fueling it?

Here are three quite contemporary situations for you to consider.

Situation number one:

> Nine-year-old Brian's parent finds a sheet of paper that he has left on the kitchen table. On the sheet Brian has listed the names of ten girls from his class and has rated each of them on the basis of appearance, intelligence and personality. None of the girls scored more than a seven on a one to ten rating scale.

Questions to consider in this situation:
- How would you feel about this situation?
- What attitudes might Brian have about girls?
- What message would you want to give Brian if he were your son?
- How would you do it?

Even parents who are trying energetically to raise their children in nonsexist ways encounter situations such as this one. Children's attitudes are also influenced by their friends, TV and society in general. It's important for Brian's parent to react to this rating sheet, but in a way that Brian can hear. Perhaps the parent could begin by asking Brian to explain the sheet and what it meant to him rather than launching into a one-way lecture. Once you understand your child's point of view and hear his explanation, it's your right and your responsibility to communicate your values. If you are disturbed that your son sees girls as objects to be rated instead of as full human beings, it's important that you communicate that to him through your words and behavior.

Situation number two:

> Mom and Dad are watching their favorite TV sitcom with their bright and curious seven-year-old daughter. The show features an attractive and charming young woman. Dad has made it clear through his nonverbal communication that he finds the young woman appealing. At a later point in the show, the attractive young woman is lying in bed waiting for her lover. Daughter turns to her dad and asks, "Do you want me to be like her?"

Questions to consider in this situation:

- What is the daughter really asking?
- What message would you want to give if you were her father? Her mother?
- How should her parents respond to communicate these messages?

It's extremely difficult as parents and educators to be aware of the messages that we communicate to children nonverbally. Yet children probably pick up more from our facial expressions and tone than they do from our words. The music, again, is more powerful than the lyrics. It appears that the daughter has noticed that Dad is very impressed with the young woman in the TV show. Daughter, even at age seven, is figuring out what kind of girl she should be now and what kind of woman she'll be when she grows up. Even if the parents clarify what they value in women, what they want their daughter to be like, she has been and will continue to be influenced by their nonverbal communication. In this case, a real situation, the daughter was quite communicative. Other children may have these questions but don't have the personality or even the language to express themselves.

Situation number three:

> A mother was shopping in a large department store with her six-year-old daughter. The daughter was quite rambunctious, constantly pulling clothes off the racks, running around, jumping, playing and talking to the other shoppers. Initially, Mom told her daughter, "Jasmine, you leave things alone. Settle down and be quiet. You're disturbing other people." Jasmine quieted down for a few minutes only to resume her activity again. Her mom finally got fed up, grabbed her firmly by the shoulders and said, "Jasmine, that's it. I did not raise you to act like this. Be quiet this instant. We're leaving and we're not going to McDonald's." Jasmine looked her mother squarely in the eyes and said, "If you don't take me to McDonalds, I'm going to tell everybody that you and Daddy were doing 'the nasty.'"

Questions to consider in this situation:

- What is the goal of Jasmine's statement to her mother?
- What message has Jasmine learned about sexual behavior?
- What would you do if you were her mother?

There's no one way to interpret this situation. It seems to me, though, that Jasmine is attempting to blackmail her mother. If her mother gives in to this, she will be encouraging her daughter's manipulation in the future. Also, it seems that Jasmine has picked up the idea that the behavior she observed between her father and mother is very bad—real blackmail material. The first question to consider is, How did Jasmine pick up this idea about her parents' behavior? She probably walked in on her parents having sex, but this has happened in many homes. Did Jasmine's parents overreact? Did they act guilty? Did they swear Jasmine to secrecy? We'll never know, but it's important to note that overreaction to an incident can leave more of an impression than the incident itself.

Let's go back to the department store. How should Jasmine's mom deal with her? Once she has handled her daughter's misbehavior, how can she

Especially for Parents

communicate to Jasmine that sex between her mom and dad is loving and good, but also private?

How Should I Respond to Advanced Sexuality Questions?

It's quite a compliment to you if your children ask you advanced questions about sexuality. They obviously feel comfortable with you and see you as a resource. It appears that your music has been sweet to their ears.

But how far should you go in answering questions such as these:

- Why don't I have a penis?
- When can I have a baby?
- How does the baby get inside the mother?
- Why do I have to have a period?
- Did you have sex when you were a teenager?
- What is a condom?
- What does it mean to be "queer."
- Why do some men want to be women?
- When are you old enough to have sex?
- How does it feel to make love?

Again there's no one right or wrong answer to these questions. Most of the guidelines listed in Chapter 3 apply to parents as well as educators. However, unlike educators who must hold back their own values, it's your right and your responsibility to communicate your values to your children. They need to know what you believe and why.

Every time your child asks you a question about sexuality it represents an opportunity for you to discuss three things: (1) values, (2) information and (3) feelings. Let's take the first question from a four year old: "Why don't I have a penis?" The parent might respond:

> "You don't have a penis because you are a girl. Girls have some body parts that boys don't have and these parts are special for girls. You have a vulva (point or touch)—that is the part of you that is covered by your underpants. Mom has a vulva, too. Vulvas are nice."

What values, information and feelings came through in that answer? How would you change the answer to reflect your own personal values and feelings?

Let's look at another question from a nine year old: "What does it mean to be queer?" This parent says:

> "Queer is one of those put-down words that some people use to talk about gay people. Gay people are men or women who have loving feelings and relationships with members of their own sex. Just like your mom and I fell in love and got married, some men fall in love with other men. Some women fall in love with other women. I don't like the word queer or fag because I know it hurts people's feelings. What do you think about that?"

What values, information and feelings came across in this answer? How would you change the answer to reflect your personal values and feelings about homosexuality?

I've given you a lot to think about in this chapter...probably more questions than answers. Here are some final messages that many parents have found helpful. I hope you'll benefit from them, as well.

Important Messages for Parents About Sexuality

1. You are the primary sex educators of your children. You are the ones who should communicate to them specific values about sexuality. Tell them what you believe and what you want for them. It's your right as well as your responsibility.
2. Your children learn about sexuality every day of their lives. They learn from their friends, TV, movies, music, from you and from society in general.
3. Don't wait for your children to ask questions about sexuality— initiate conversations. Use everyday occurrences (watching TV, diapering a baby) to begin conversations about sexuality.

4. You can be effective sexuality educators, even though that role may seem difficult or uncomfortable at first.
5. You don't have to be an expert or completely at ease with the topic of sexuality to do a good job of educating your children about sex.
6. You communicate with your children about sexuality both verbally and nonverbally. Your children are aware of what you do and don't say, your reactions and your behavior. Try to make sure that your actions are consistent with the values you hope to teach your children.
7. Although it's best to start talking to your children about sexuality when they are very young, it's never too late to start.
8. If your children ask questions, don't worry about whether they are too young to know the answers. Children understand what they are ready to understand. However, answer at your child's level of understanding and ask for feedback to determine what he or she has understood. Remember, every question is an opportunity to discuss values, information and feelings.
9. Listen attentively to your children. Let them know that you care about their feelings and respect their ideas—even if you don't agree with them.
10. Use your sense of humor when talking about sexuality. Most conversations need not be serious. Children often complain that their parents are too long-winded and too serious.
11. Have a variety of books, pamphlets, and other resources available around the house—some that you can give to your children, some that they can pick to read, and some that you would find helpful in answering your own questions.
12. It's good to touch and hug your children and show love, regardless of how old they are.
13. Remember, education about sexuality is a life-long process, not something that will be accomplished in one conversation.
14. Don't forget the music!

Appendix A

Sexuality Concepts in Concrete Terms

These explanations have been developed for primary students, ages four to seven. They demonstrate examples of "less" answers that break down complicated ideas for concrete thinking children.

Adoption

1. Sometimes a mom and dad have a baby and they realize they can't give it the love, food, shelter and clothing it needs.
2. If the mom and dad can find another man and woman to be this child's legal parents, the child is adopted.
3. Once children are adopted, they're members of their new family forever, just like all other sons and daughters.

Childbirth

1. Babies grow inside their mothers in a special place called the uterus.
2. The baby *usually* comes out of the mother's body through an opening between her legs (called the vagina).
3. But sometimes the doctor makes a cut (or an opening) in the mom's abdomen (point to it) and takes the baby out that way.
4. Either way that the baby is born is OK.

Clitoris

1. The clitoris is a special part of a girl's body.
2. The clitoris is a very small body part between a girl's legs.
3. When the clitoris is touched, it usually brings good feelings.

Erection

1. Sometimes a boy's or a man's penis gets stiff.
2. It's something that happens to penises from time to time and it's OK.
3. It often means the boy is having a good feeling in his penis.

Intercourse

1. Intercourse is something people do when they're grown up.
2. It happens when a man puts his penis inside the woman's vagina.
3. People have intercourse for a lot of different reasons.
4. One reason is to make a baby; another reason is to show love and get good feelings.

Life Cycle

1. When you're first born, you are a baby.
2. As you grow and change, you become a child, then a teenager, then an adult.
3. Adults get older—like some of your grandparents—and then all people die at some point.
4. The time that we spend growing and changing from birth to death is called the life cycle.

Menstruation

1. Menstruation, or having periods, is something that happens to girls when they get older.
2. It helps make a girl's body able to have babies.
3. It's something natural and healthy that all girls experience.

Penis

1. The penis is the body part of a man or boy that hangs between his legs.
2. The penis is very sensitive and usually feels good when it is touched.
3. A boy uses his penis to urinate or "pee" and for sexual intercourse when he grows up.

Reproduction

1. Reproduction means to make more.
2. With living things, it means to make more of the same kind of living thing...more dogs (puppies), cats (kittens) or humans (babies).

Uterus

1. The uterus is the place inside a woman's body where the baby grows before it's born.
2. The uterus is inside the woman's body, just below her belly button.

Vagina

1. The vagina is an opening between a woman's legs.
2. A baby comes out through this opening when it's born.
3. The penis goes into this opening during sexual intercourse.

Disability

1. All human beings are alike in some ways and different in some ways.
2. Some differences you can see and some you can't see.
3. Some people have a difference that makes it hard for them to do certain things.
4. For example, they may have trouble walking, hearing, writing or understanding things.
5. No matter what differences we have, we all have the same need to be loved, to have friends and to have fun.

Appendix B

Organizations Involved in Sexuality Education

American Association of Sex Educators, Counselors, and Therapists
435 North Michigan Avenue, Suite 1717
Chicago, IL 60611
(312) 644-0828

A membership organization that sponsors training workshops and an annual conference, and publishes a newsletter and journal. Also certifies sex educators, counselors and therapists.

Center for Population Options
1025 Vermont Street N.W., Suite 210
Washington, DC 20005
(202) 347-5700

A private, non-profit organization committed to the reduction of teenage pregnancy in the United States. CPO conducts research, develops and pilot-tests resource materials, and provides technical assistance and training. Publishes the *Life Planning Education* curriculum. Acts as an advocate to influence public policy regarding teenage pregnancy, sexuality messages in the media and AIDS. Publishes resources for AIDS educators and conducts conferences on AIDS and adolescents.

Children's Defense Fund
122 C Street, N.W.
Washington, DC 20001
(202) 628-8787

A private, non-profit child advocacy organization that focuses on programs and policies affecting large numbers of children. CDF's pregnancy prevention efforts include: (1) raising the public's awareness of the problems; (2) disseminating information about research and effective outreach and service approaches; (3) advocating public policy initiatives; and (4) examining the role of the media and the messages it gives youth, especially minority youth. CDF Adolescent Pregnancy Prevention Clearinghouse publishes excellent bimonthly reports on timely issues in the field.

ETR Associates (Education, Training, Research)
P.O. Box 1830
Santa Cruz, CA 95061-1830
(408) 438-4081

A private consulting group that conducts sexuality education, teacher training and research in California and around the country. Its publishing division, Network Publications, develops and distributes family life and sexuality education resources, including curricula, training manuals, booklets and pamphlets. Publishes a quarterly journal, *Family Life Educator*.

New Jersey Network for Family Life Education
Center for Community Education
B4087 Kilmer Campus
Rutgers School of Social Work
New Brunswick, NJ 08903
(201) 932-7798

A coalition of public and private non-profit agencies joined in their support of including family life education—and specifically instruction about human sexuality—as an integral part of the New Jersey public school program. Provides a resource center, workshops and networking opportunities. The newsletter, *Family Life Matters*, contains practical ideas and information useful to all family life educators.

Planned Parenthood Federation of America
810 Seventh Avenue
New York, NY 10019
(212) 541-7800

The national organization that provides leadership to local Planned Parenthood affiliates around the country. Disseminates information and resources to be used in sexuality education and pregnancy prevention programs, including pamphlets, flipcharts and videos.

Sex Education Coalition of Metropolitan Washington
P.O. Box 3101
Silver Spring, MD 20901
(301) 593-8557

A membership organization that promotes positive sexuality education in the Washington metropolitan area and in the nation. Offers low-cost workshops and training, an annual media fair, free film loans, a quarterly newsletter, as well as pamphlets and curricula.

Sex Information and Education Council of the U.S. (SIECUS)
130 W. 42nd Street, Suite 2500
New York, NY 10036
(212) 819-9770

A private, nonprofit membership organization that advocates for human sexuality and provides information and education on sexual matters through a clearinghouse and resource center. Publishes a variety of resource guides, bibliographies and the *SIECUS Report*, a bimonthly newsletter.

The following organizations distribute low-cost workbooks, coloring books and pamphlets on family life education topics for children:

Channing L. Bete Co.
200 State Road
South Deerfield, MA 01273-0200
(800) 628-7733

Equal Justice Consultants
Educational Products
P.O. Box 583
Eugene, OR 97405

Hammett
2393 Vauxhall Road
Union, NJ 07083
(800) 672-1932

Milliken Publishing Company
Rodman Associates
P.O. Box 354
Horsham, PA 19044

Opportunities for Learning, Inc.
20417 Nordhoff Street, Dept. 3N
Chatsworth, CA 91311

Appendix C

Books for Professionals, Parents and Children

Books for Professionals

Bernstein, Anne. 1980. *The Flight of the Stork*. New York: Dell Publishing Co.

Identifies six different stages that children ages three to twelve experience as they develop their cognitive understanding of procreation. Emphasizes that parents should be aware of their children's level of understanding when discussing the different aspects of pregnancy and birth.

Brick, Peggy, et al. 1989. *Bodies, Birth and Babies: Sexuality Education in Early Childhood Programs*. Hackensack, NJ: The Center for Family Life Education Planned Parenthood of Bergen County, Inc.

Tells how schools can take responsibility for their role in promoting the sexual learning of young children. Recommends 12 learning strategies early childhood educators can use to help develop sexual health and self-esteem in young children.

Center for Early Adolescence. 1980. *Early Adolescent Sexuality: Resources for Parents, Professionals and Young People*. Carrboro, NC: Center for Early Adolescence.

An extensive bibliography of general reading materials, journals and periodicals, training materials, curricula and films related to early adolescent sexuality.

Derman-Sparks, Louise and the A.B.C. Task Force. 1989. *Anti-Bias Curriculum: Tools for Empowering Young Children.* Washington, DC: National Association for the Education of Young Children.

Excellent and inexpensive tool for creating educational environments and curricula that encourage acceptance of human differences and discourage bias. Contains a wealth of practical advice and checklists for eliminating bias in educational programs.

DeSpelder, Lynne Anne and Albert Lee Stricklin. 1982. *Family Life Education: Resources for the Elementary Classroom—Grades 4, 5 and 6.* Santa Cruz, CA: ETR Associates/Network Publications.

Over 75 activities on a variety of topics to be used in health and family life education classes for elementary school children. Includes age-appropriate discussions of human sexuality, and reproducible diagrams and worksheets.

Goldman, Ronald and Juliette Goldman. 1982. *Children's Sexual Thinking.* Boston: Routledge and Kegan Paul.

Reports on interviews with hundreds of children ages five to fifteen in North America, England, Sweden and Australia. Examines how children perceive aging, parental roles, gender identity, sex roles, conception and birth, contraception, marriage and nudity. Cites implications of findings for sex education.

Healy, Jane M. 1987. *Your Child's Growing Mind: A Parent's Guide to Learning from Birth to Adolescence.* New York: Doubleday.

Gives a synopsis of cognitive development at different stages of childhood. Offers advice for promoting children's capacity to learn and understand abstract concepts. A good resource for professionals.

Irvington Public Schools. 1990. *Family Life Education Curriculum Guide: Volume I, K-6*. Irvington, NJ.

Identifies a scope and sequence for family life education in grades kindergarten through six and in special education. Lists appropriate content for each grade level and a brief description of possible activities. Also contains descriptions of teacher training and a list of print and audiovisual resources for the elementary classroom.

Mendler, Allen N. *Smiling at Yourself: Educating Young Children About Stress and Self-Esteem.* 1990. Santa Cruz, CA: ETR Associates/Network Publications.

Written to assist children in understanding what stress is and what they can do about it. Filled with activities that teach problem solving, positive imagery and relaxation techniques. Provides adults with practical steps to help children develop an "I can do it" attitude.

Quackenbush, Marcia and Sylvia Villarreal. 1988. *Does AIDS Hurt?: Educating Young Children About AIDS.* Santa Cruz, CA: ETR Associates/ Network Publications.

An excellent guidebook for educating young children about AIDS. Emphasizes the use of age-appropriate responses to children's questions, maintaining that young children don't need explicit information about AIDS. Underscores the importance of a solid general health education to give children the tools to understand concepts about disease transmission.

Roberts, Elizabeth J. *Childhood Sexual Learning: The Unwritten Curriculum.* 1980. Cambridge, MA: Ballinger Publishing.

Explores the many areas in which learning about sexuality takes place, including the family, school, television, social services, peer groups and religion. Examines the assumptions about sexuality that form the foundation of institutional policies and practices.

Books for Parents

Calderone, Mary and Eric Johnson. 1981. *The Family Book About Sexuality.* New York: Harper & Row.

Relevant to parents of children of all ages. Besides stressing the importance of sexuality education within the home, the book provides an extensive glossary, a bibliography listing additional readings and a list of agencies specializing in sexuality-related issues.

Calderone, Mary and James Ramey. 1982. *Talking with Your Child About Sex: Questions and Answers for Children From Birth to Puberty.* New York: Ballantine Books.

Provides an overview of questions that may be asked by children at various stages from childhood to puberty. Answers are provided to help parents respond to their children's concerns.

Gochros, Jean. *What to Say After You Clear Your Throat: A Parent's Guide to Sex Education.* 1980. Oahu, HI: Press Pacifica.

Discusses the art of communicating about sexuality. Provides a great deal of practical information, such as strategies for beginning conversations about sexuality and techniques for handling troublesome home situations. Includes a special section on sexuality education with disabled people.

Goldman, Ronald and Juliette Goldman. 1987. *Show Me Yours! Understanding Children's Sexuality.* New York: Doubleday.

Examines what children know and don't know about sexuality, gender and reproduction. The authors' research in five countries suggests that much of childrens' ignorance stems from their parents' inhibition and from inadequate school programs.

Gordon, Sol and Judith Gordon. 1983. *Raising a Child Conservatively in a Sexually Permissive World.* New York: Simon & Schuster.

Includes chapters on coming to terms with your own sexuality, becoming an "askable" parent, self-esteem, the role of the schools and questions most frequently asked by parents and children, along with suggested responses. Written with warmth and concern.

Morris, L.B. *Talking Sex with Your Kids.* 1984. New York: Simon & Schuster.

Serves as a handbook that provides answers for parents who wonder when they should discuss sexuality with their children and what they should say. Easy to read.

Pogrebin, Letty C. *Growing Up Free: Raising Your Child in the '80's.* 1980. New York: McGraw Hill, Inc.

Covers child-rearing from conception to maturity. Emphasizes non-sexist sexuality education and parenting. Highly recommended for both parents and professionals.

Ratner, Marilyn and Susan Chamlin. 1985. *Straight Talk: Sexuality for Parents and Kids 4-7.* Westchester, PA: Planned Parenthood of Westchester, Inc.

A short, very practical book for parents. Layout is attractive and easy to read. Includes answers to questions that young children commonly ask about sexuality.

Sex Information and Education Council of the U.S. 1983. *Oh No! What Do I Do Now?* New York: SIECUS.

A wonderful pamphlet that helps parents decide in advance about the sexuality messages they want to give their children. Helps parents practice responses to anticipated questions and behavior. Also available in Spanish.

Appendix C

Somers, Leon and Barbara C. Somers. 1989. *Talking to Your Children About Love and Sex*. Ontario, Canada: New American Library.

Teaches parents how to convey to their children the acceptance and sensitivity that helps instill healthy attitudes about love and sex.

Wattleton, Faye. *How to Talk With Your Child About Sexuality: A Parent's Guide*. 1986. Garden City, NJ: Doubleday.

A how-to book that explains how children interpret sexual information. Stresses the importance of talking with sons as well as daughters and recommends actions parents can take in specific situations.

Books for Young Children

Andry, Andrew and Steven Schepp. 1974. *How Babies Are Made*. Boston, MA: Little, Brown & Co., Inc.

Includes discussions and colorful illustrations of reproduction among animals, plants and humans. Simply written with clear pictures. Factually accurate and up-to-date. Most appropriate for children who already understand the concept of human reproduction.

Brenner, Barbara. 1973. *Bodies*. New York: E.P. Dutton.

Uses multicultural photographs of children, some of whom are nude, to give a positive perspective on the uniqueness of each human body. Although the book is dated, its "music" is nice.

Brooks, Robert. 1983. *So That's How I Was Born*. New York: Simon & Schuster.

Relates factual information about basic reproduction, using language a young child can understand. Includes watercolor drawings of racially diverse children. Deals with human reproduction within a family context.

Cole, Joanna. 1984. *How You Were Born*. New York: William Morrow & Co., Inc.

Relates the story of birth in a simple, informative manner. Designed for parents to read to their children. Includes actual photography of the developing fetus inside the womb.

Gordon, Sol and Judith Gordon. 1982. *Did the Sun Shine Before You Were Born?* Revised Edition. Fayetteville, NY: Ed-U-Press.

Intended for parents to read to their preschool or primary school-age children. Keeping their focus on family living, the authors answer the classic question, "Where do babies come from?" clearly and concisely. This book includes artful drawings of children and families of different races. Describes different kinds of families. Explains the birth process in terms that preschoolers can understand.

Gordon, Sol. 1979. *Girls Are Girls and Boys Are Boys...So What's the Difference?* Fayetteville, NY: Ed-U-Press.

Encourages boys and girls to be anything they want to be and to disregard the limitations of traditional sex roles. Discusses male and female bodies and how they change at puberty. Although the book could be read to younger children, it is more appropriate for children ages seven to ten who can understand the subtle humor used to explain gender roles. Drawings depict children of all ethnic groups.

Gruenberg, Sidonie M. 1973. *The Wonderful Story of How You Were Born*. New York: Doubleday.

Describes how life begins and how a baby develops from the union of an egg and a sperm. Compares a variety of parents (animals and humans) and describes the growth and maturation of humans.

Levine, Milton and Jean Seligman. 1978. *A Baby Is Born*. Revised Edition. New York: Golden Press.

Gives information about animal and human reproduction in a simple manner. Explains reproduction, multiple births, the importance of breastfeeding and how babies grow and develop. Drawings of families of many races add to the appeal of this book.

Mayle, Peter. 1973. *Where Did I Come From?* New York: Lyle Stuart.

Answers the question "Where did I come from?" in a humorous style that young children will enjoy, but may not fully understand. Illustrated with chubby human cartoon characters. Explains intercourse, reproductive organs, pregnancy and birth. Uses analogies that might be confusing for young children who tend to take things literally. A popular book that can be used best by parents who read selected passages for their children.

Nilsson, Leonard. 1975. *How Was I Born? A Photographic Story of Reproduction and Birth for Children*. New York: Delacorte Press.

Uses extraordinary photography of fetal development and warm family scenes to tell the story of reproduction and birth. Designed for parents to read to their children.

Sheffield, Margaret and Sheila Bewley. 1973. *Where Do Babies Come From?* New York: Alfred A. Knopf, Inc.

Offers young children a clear description of reproduction and birth.

Waxman, Stephanie. 1979. *Growing Up—Feeling Good: A Child's Introduction to Sexuality*. Los Angeles, CA: Panjandrum Books.

An excellent introduction to many important concepts about human sexuality. Presented with simplicity and dignity.

Books for Puberty-Age Children

Betancourt, Jeanne. 1983. *Am I Normal? An Illustrated Guide to Your Changing Body* and *Dear Diary: An Illustrated Guide to Your Changing Body*. New York: Avon Books.

Based on the award-winning films of the same titles by Debra Franco and David Shepard. The first title depicts Jimmy's successful efforts to learn, from a variety of sources, the truth about boys' sexual development. The second title describes two weeks in the life of Jamie, during which she comes to understand the normalcy of her own body and internal time clock.

Gardner-Loulan, Joann, Bonnie Lopez and Marcia Quackenbush. 1981. *Period*. San Francisco, CA: Volcano Press.

A unique book which addresses the concerns that most young women have about menstruating and other topics such as hair and weight. Down-to-earth, readable style that is warm and appealing. Encourages readers to recognize that individual differences related to menstruation and development are natural and normal. Spanish edition, *Periodo,* also available.

Gitchel, Sam and Lorri Foster. 1985. *Let's Talk About...s-e-x: A Read and Discuss Guide for People 9 to 12 and Their Parents*. Fresno, CA: Planned Parenthood of Central California.

Introduction for parents that covers how much children need to know, good times to talk and practical suggestions for talking to children about sex. Main text for preteens and parents to read together. Covers facts and feelings about puberty, sexual intercourse and reproduction. Spanish/English bilingual edition available under the title *Hablemos Acerca del... s-e-x-o: Un Libro Para Toda La Familia Acerca De La Pubertad.*

Gordon, Sol. 1983. *Facts About Sex for Today's Youth*. Revised Edition. Fayetteville, NY: Ed-U-Press.

Provides an overview of sexuality for teenagers. Briefly discusses reproduction, love, premarital sex, male and female anatomy, sex differences and other topics. Clear and factual drawings and graphics. Discourages adolescent sexual intercourse. Well illustrated.

Johnson, Eric. 1985. *Love and Sex in Plain Language.* Revised Edition. New York: Harper & Row.

Discusses reproduction, heredity, fetal development, birth, sex differences, sexual intercourse, birth control, venereal disease, dating and love in language that is easily understood by most teenagers. Available in most public libraries.

Mayle, Peter. 1979. *What's Happening to Me?* New York: Lyle Stuart.

Tells the story of puberty with humorous illustrations. Emphasizes individual differences—ages for reaching puberty, breast size and penis size. Presents information about such topics as erections, wet dreams and menstruation in a liberal manner. Usually well received by pre- and early adolescents. Available in most book stores.

Madaras, Lynda and Area Madaras. 1983. *The What's Happening to My Body? Book for Girls.* New York: Newmarket Press.

Provides a wonderful opportunity for mothers (and fathers, too) to help their daughters ages nine to thirteen understand and celebrate their sexuality and their individuality.

Madaras, Lynda and Area Madaras. 1987. *Lynda Madaras' Growing-Up Guide for Girls.* New York: Newmarket Press.

An innovative workbook/journal for girls ages nine to fifteen, which combines conversational text with quizzes, exercises, checklists, illustrations, anecdotes and personal stories.

Madaras, Lynda and Dane Saavedra. 1984. *The What's Happening to My Body? Book for Boys.* New York: Newmarket Press.

For preteen boys to read on their own or with their parents to understand the physical and emotional changes of puberty.

Palmer, Pat. 1977. *The Mouse, the Monster and Me.* San Luis Obispo, CA: Impact Publishers, Inc.

A good resource for teaching upper elementary students about the need for assertiveness skills. Presents techniques that children can understand and use.

References

Bernstein, Anne. 1980. *The flight of the stork.* New York: Dell Publishing Company, Inc.

Clark, Sam, Laurie Zabin and Janet Hardy. 1984. Sex, contraception and parenthood: Experience and attitudes among urban black young men. *Family Planning Perspectives* 16(2): 77-82.

Derman-Sparks, Louise and the A.B.C. Task Force. 1989. *Anti-bias curriculum: Tools for empowering young children.* Washington, DC: National Association for the Education of Young Children.

Derman-Sparks, Louise, Maria Gutierrez and Carol B. Phillips. 1990. *Teaching young children to resist bias: What parents can do.* Washington, DC: National Association for the Education of Young Children.

Fraiberg, Selma. 1959. *The magic years.* New York: Charles Scribner & Sons.

Gochros, Jean. 1980. *What to say after you clear your throat.* Kailua, HI: Press Pacifica.

Ianni, Francis. 1989. The search for structure: A report on American youth today. New York: The Free Press.

Maccoby, Eleanor. 1990. Gender and relationships: A developmental account. *American Psychologist* 45 (4): 513-520.

The Touch Film. 1983. Sterling Productions, 1112 N. Ridgeland, Oak Park, IL 60302, (312) 383-1710, 16mm, 22 min.

About the Author

Pamela M. Wilson is a nationally known program consultant and trainer in the areas of sexuality education, youth development, parent-child communication, adolescent pregnancy and parenting, and prejudice reduction. For much of her career she has led sexuality education programs with children of all ages and with parents. She has also trained educators and counselors throughout the country.

Ms. Wilson, a social worker by training, is past president of the Sex Education Coalition of Metropolitan Washington, a board member of the Sex Information and Education Council of the United States (SIECUS) and an A.A.S.E.C.T. certified sexuality educator. She has coauthored other sexuality education publications including *Families Talk About Sexuality*, a curriculum distributed by the American Association for Counseling and Development, and *Sexuality Education: A Resource Book*, published by Network Publications.

THE THINGS CHILDREN ASK!
Get The Answers You Need From Our Critical Issues Series

These practical handbooks help you discuss many sensitive topics with children up to age ten!

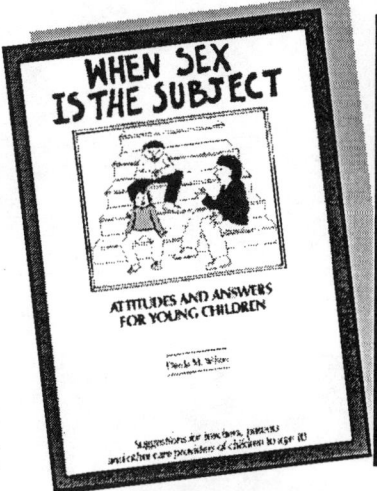

When Sex is the Subject:
Attitudes and Answers
for Young Children
99 pgs./paper, $14.95

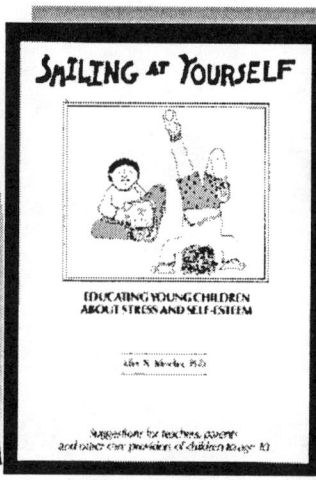

Smiling At Yourself:
Educating Young Children About Stress
and Self-Esteem
150 pgs./paper, $14.95

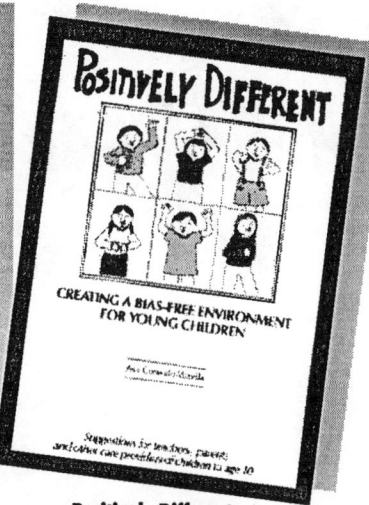

Positively Different:
Creating a Bias-Free
Environment for Young Children
93 pgs./paper, $14.95

These are just a few of the helpful titles in this bestselling series!

Additional titles cover personal health, family life, mental and emotional health, disease prevention and control, substance abuse prevention and more! Each accessible handbook helps you:

- **Learn Sensitive, Age-Appropriate Responses to Children's Health-Related Questions**
- **Make Complex Terms Simple and Easy to Understand for Children**
- **Take Advantage of Spontaneous, Teachable Moments**
- **Improve Adult/Child Communication Skills**
- **Benefit From the Experience of Leading Experts**

For More Information and a Complete Catalog of Over 500 Family Life and Health Education Books, Videos and Pamphlets...

Call Toll-Free 1 (800) 321-4407

or contact:

ETR Associates/Network Publications
Sales Department
P.O. Box 1830
Santa Cruz, CA 95061-1830
FAX: (408) 438-4284